# Otoacoustic Emissions

*Basic Science and Clinical Applications*

**A Singular Audiology Text**
Jeffrey L. Danhauer, Ph.D.
Audiology Editor

# Otoacoustic Emissions

*Basic Science and Clinical Applications*

Edited by

## Charles I. Berlin, Ph.D.

*Kenneth & Frances Barnes Bullington Professor of Hearing Science*
*Professor and Director*
*Kresge Hearing Research Laboratory of the South*
*Department of Otorhinolaryngology and Biocommunication*
*Louisiana State University Medical School*
*New Orleans, Louisiana*

## National Organization for Hearing Research

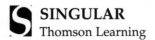

SINGULAR
Thomson Learning

Africa • Australia • Canada • Denmark • Japan • Mexico • New Zealand • Philippines
Puerto Rico • Singapore • Spain • United Kingdom • United States

## NOTICE TO THE READER

Publisher does not warrant or guarantee any of the products described herein or perform any independent analysis in connection with any of the product information contained herein. Publisher does not assume, and expressly disclaims, any obligation to obtain and include information other than that provided to it by the manufacturer.

The reader is expressly warned to consider and adopt all safety precautions that might be indicated by the activities herein and to avoid all potential hazards. By following the instructions contained herein, the reader willingly assumes all risks in connection with such instructions.

The Publisher makes no representation or warranties of any kind, including but not limited to, the warranties of fitness for particular purpose or merchantability, nor are any such representations implied with respect to the material set forth herein, and the publisher takes no responsibility with respect to such material. The publisher shall not be liable for any special, consequential, or exemplary damages resulting, in whole or part, from the readers' use of, or reliance upon, this material.

Library of Congress Cataloging-in-Publication Data:
ISBN: 1-5659-3619-1

# Contents

# Contributors

**Carolina Abdala, Ph.D.**
Assistant Scientist
House Ear Institute
Los Angeles, California

**Charles I. Berlin, Ph.D.**
Kenneth and Francis Bullington
Professor of Hearing Science
Director
Kresge Hearing Research Laboratory
of the South
Department of Otorhinolaryngology
and Biocommunication
Louisiana State University Medical
School
New Orleans, Louisiana

**Richard P. Bobbin, Ph.D.**
Professor
Lousiana State University Medical
Center
New Orleans, Louisiana

**Chu Chen, Ph.D.**
Department of Otorhinolaryngology
and Biocommunication
Lousianna State University Medical
Center
New Orleans, Louisiana

**Linda J. Hood, Ph.D.**
Associate Professor
Kresge Hearing Research Laboratory
Louisiana State University Medical
Center
New Orleans, Louisiana

**Jer-Min Huang, M.D., Ph.D.**
Assistant Professor
Louisiana State University
Medical Center
New Orleans, Louisiana

**Bronya J. B. Keats, Ph.D.**
Professor
Department of Biometry and Genetics
Acting Head of the Center of Excellence
of Molecular Human Genetics
Louisiana State University Medical
Center
New Orleans, Louisiana

**David T. Kemp**
Institute of Laryngology and Otology
University College London
London, England

**Kevin H. Knuth, Ph.D.**
Research Associate
Dynamic Brain Imaging Laboratory
Albert Einstein College of Medicine
Bronx, New York

**Shu-Tze Lin, M.P.H.**
Department of Otorhinolaryngology
and Biocommunication
Louisiana State University Medical
Center
New Orleans, Louisiana

**David M. Mills, Ph.D.**
Virginia Merrill Bloedel Hearing
Research Center
Department of Otolaryngology, Head
and Neck Surgery
University of Washington
Seattle, Washington

**Matthew Money, M.D.**
Department of Otorhinolaryngology
and Biocommunication
Louisiana State University Medical
Center
New Orleans, Louisiana

**Anastas P. Nenov, M.D., Ph.D.**
Department of Otorhinolaryngology
and Biocommuncation
Louisiana State University Medical
Center
New Orleans, Louisiana

**Yvonne S. Sininger, Ph.D.**
Director
Children's Auditory Research and
Evaluation Center
House Ear Institute
Los Angeles, California

**Ruth A. Skellet, Ph.D.**
Department of Otorhinolaryngology
and Biocommunication
Louisiana State University Medical
Center
New Orleans, Louisiana

# Foreword

This is the third book in what has become an exciting yearly endeavor for our staff as well as Singular Publishing Group, and represents the crowning presentation of a Hearing Science trilogy. The first book in the series was *Hair Cells and Hearing Aids* honoring **Dr. William Brownell's** revolutionary discovery of outer hair cell motility, and the second was *Neurotransmission and Hearing Loss* honoring **Dr. Robert Wenthold's** germinal and critical work in small amino acids as transmitters in both the cochlea and the auditory nervous system. Both Brownell's compendium and this one on *Otoacoustic Emissions* contain unique teaching media in the form of compact discs. But to fully appreciate the scope of the science honored here, we urge the serious reader to study all three books as examples of celebrations of work which has changed the course of our science.

The 1996 scientific meeting was indeed stimulating and exciting to the nearly 100 people attending. After introductory remarks by our **Chancellor, Dr. Mervin Trail**, and our **Department Head, Dr. Daniel W. Nuss**, **Dr. Douglas Webster** introduced the featured speaker.

**Dr. David Kemp** began with a scholarly and historical clarification of the little appreciated role **Dr. T. Gold** played in the 1940s when Gold predicted the now well-accepted notion of an active process in the cochlea. One of Dr. Gold's contemporaries was Dr. Georg von Békèsy, who ultimately won the Nobel Prize for his work on cadaver cochleas. It was Gold who argued on theoretical and psychophysical grounds that there had to be an active process in the cochlea, but von Békèsy's empirical physiological data prevailed and the active process was consequently ignored for many years. Attempts by the respected English scientist-physician **Lionel Naftalin, M.D.** to revive thinking about an active amplifier which he felt might reside in (unconfirmed) piezo-electrical properties of the tectorial membrane also fell on "deaf ears." Dr. Kemp, who began his scientific career as a geophysicist, clearly had special empathy for this misdirection. In part because of his unorthodox path into hearing science, the importance of his own work was not immediately appreciated until many years after its initial publication; *Nature* in fact rejected it on grounds that it was of mostly clinical interest, and clinicians of course failed to recognize the significance of the findings at the time.

His (perhaps too kind) assessment of the short-sightedness of peers who ignored, belittled, and criticized his and Gold's theories and discoveries, and his gentle but realistic critique of reviewers and equipment manufacturers were to me exemplary. His commentary will bring a sense of déjà vu and vindication to scientific authors who have ever had papers rejected and to our own kindred of writers of "approved but not funded" grants. I have always wondered, perhaps cynically, if granting agencies kept records of great discoveries their reviewers rejected at first. It is no wonder that the history of information dissemination in science often highlights the importance of perseverance as much as rigor.

During his extemporaneous presentation Dr. Kemp used a laptop computer to display dynamic models of cochlear echoes which I found particularly stimulating and which clarified for me many of the elusive principles of echo generation. **Kemp's** truly brilliant oral presentation was matched only by the clarity and scope of the chapter he submitted for his contribution. I anticipate that this chapter and the accompanying CD will become required reading for students of the ear and hearing for years to come. **I know we, and our students, will learn from these demonstrations and examples on the enclosed CD-ROM which Kemp kindly prepared especially for this book.** His conclusions painted a fascinating scenario for where we might go in the future with his important discovery.

Dr. Kemp commented on the problems many clinicians have with the mathematics of otoacoustic emissions and lauded the mathematical tutorial written by **Dr. Kevin Knuth** which is given at the end of this book; Dr. Kemp also predicted that future clinically practical instruments will study many more distortion products than the most commonly assessed $2f_1$–$f_2$.

A poster session of contributed papers on otoacoustic emissions featuring works by **Philip Noel, M.D., and Peter Rigby, M.D.** among others preceded the next talk by Dr. Bobbin.

**Dr. Richard P. Bobbin** then presented new work on his own behalf and that of **Chu Chen, Ph.D., Anastas Nenov, M.D., and Ruth Skellett, Ph.D.**, his collaborators. They presented exciting new ideas on ATP as a neurotransmitter involved in the quadratic distortion product; this work built upon important observations that Dr. Bobbin and his team, led in this instance by **Sharon Kujawa, Ph.D.**, have already made about the quadratic distortion product. Drs. Huang, Xie, and Hickham and I in the laboratory are intrigued with, and are publishing on, the quadratic distortion product in no small measure because its time course is quite different from the $2f_1$–$f_2$ (cubic) distortion product and may reflect as yet undiscovered mechanisms in the cochlea.

A luncheon presenting the award was held after Dr. Bobbin's talk. **The $5,000 prize was presented to Dr. Kemp, and, in his respect for the goals of supporting research and supporting our laboratory, he and his wife Gillian contributed the prize back into Kam's Fund! It was a gracious and magnanimous act, typical of the man who has given so much and** asked for so little in return from his colleagues. Dr. Kemp, please accept another expression of our gratitude and respect for your many acts of kindness and scientific collegiality and our special congratulations for this landmark chapter marking the 20th anniversary of the publication of your discovery.

Dr. David Mills, representing the Bloedel Center in Seattle, Washington, presented his important original work on two components of Distortion Product Emissions, based on the principle that the active process and the passive process in the cochlea support different parts of the DPOAE.

Dr. Yvonne Sininger presented her work and represented her colleague Dr. Carolina Abdala in reporting on new and exciting data on Distortion Products in Infants and Children. Some of Dr. Kemp's chapter-based comments on tuning curves and distortion product sources talk to these issues directly.

Dr. Jer-Min Huang, who is an otolaryngologist and audiologist and also holds a Ph.D. in Physiology, represented Drs. Keats, Money, and Ms. Linn in describing his work on using DPOAE's for Genetic Phenotyping in deaf and normal hearing mice. It was this collaboration, led by Dr. Bronya J. B. Keats, that located the *dn/dn* gene for recessive deafness on Chromosome 19 of the mouse. ( Keats, B. J. B., Nouri, N., Huang, J-M., Money, M., Webster, D. B., and Berlin, C. I. The deafness locus (*dn*) maps to mouse Chromosome 19. *Mammalian Genome, 6,* 8-10. 1995.)

Finally, Dr. Linda J. Hood, 1994 President of the American Academy of Audiology, showed how emissions might be used to identify human carriers of genes for recessive deafness.

During this period of our scientific endeavors, **Dr. Kevin Knuth**, a physicist, was a postdoctoral fellow in our lab; in teaching the necessary math and physics to some of our students, he hit upon the idea of preparing a tutorial for this volume. It is presented as an Appendix for the special use of teachers who might be using this book as a text for their students and earned special mention from Dr. Kemp himself.

### *Our gratitude to three special supporters of our work*

**Rona Becker Mirmelstein** died in November of 1992, before any of the books, or the symposia on which they were based, were begun. She and I discussed this concept many times, of using her gift to start a Scientific Prize and a Meeting to precede her beloved Gala. Her legacy of respect for Hearing Research and the Kresge Laboratory will live forever in these volumes and in the concept of recognizing and rewarding the world's outstanding hearing scientists for their intellectual contributions to the welfare of mankind. **We hope in the future to be able to establish a Professorship in her name which will fund these scientific presentations in perpetuity.**

This year, the publication honoring **Dr. David Kemp's** 20th Anniversary of the report of Otoacoustic Emissions has been underwritten by **Dr. Geraldine Fox** of the National Organization for Hearing Research. **Dr. Fox** was described in our most recent Gala program as

> the foremost lay citizen in the United States personally responsible for the separation of Communication Disorders from the Neurology Institute and the subsequent formation of the National Institute of Deafness and other Communication Disorders (NIDCD). Her legendary work with Senator Harkin and Representative Claude Pepper in establishing the NIDCD, despite many real and imagined obstacles, has become a roadmap for private citizens interested in changing how our government works. Dr. Fox, married to Richard Fox of Philadelphia, is now the President of her own National Organization for Hearing Research, a Philanthropic organization which supports the Kresge Lab as well as many other similar research organizations throughout the country.

We commend her once again for her vision and her philanthropic spirit.

Finally, a new star has stepped forward to support us in a different way. She is **Frances Barnes Bullington**, a former speech pathologist and widow of **Kenneth Bullington. Kenneth Bullington** was himself a celebrated engineer for the Bell Laboratories whose work on ultra-high frequency radio waves supported the Distant Early Warning Line that protected our country during the Cold War. It is noteworthy that so much in the way of geophysical and engineering talent is being celebrated here in the persons of Gold, Kemp, and Bullington.

**Mrs. Bullington** has donated generously to the **LSUMC Foundation**, endowing a Professorship on my behalf, which allows me to sign this Foreword for the first time as ...

**Charles I. Berlin, Ph.D.**
**The First Kenneth and Frances Barnes Bullington**
**Professor of Hearing Science**
**and**
**Director of the Kresge Hearing Research Laboratory of the South**
**Professor, Departments of Otorhinolaryngology and**
**Biocommunication, Physiology and Communication Disorders**

**LSU Medical Center**
**October 12, 1997. New Orleans, Louisiana**

# OTOACOUSTIC EMISSIONS
## Distorted Echoes of the Cochlea's Travelling Wave

*David T. Kemp*

Institute of Laryngology and Otology,
University College London,

This book coincides with the 20th anniversary of the identification of otoacoustic emissions (OAEs). OAEs are both a fascinating auditory phenomenon and an important tool for auditory investigation and research. Remarkably it is also just 50 years since Thomas Gold published his revolutionary ideas about amplification in the cochlea and since he made his prediction of spontaneous acoustic emissions from the disordered ear (Gold, 1948).

In this chapter I provide a broad review of what OAEs really are, what they relate to, and where we are going with them. This is not a review of the now vast OAE literature, but more of an anniversary celebration. It is an attempt to reintroduce some important OAE topics and concepts and to balance the partial accounts that inevitably accompany the introduction of new commercial technology.

Otoacoustic emissions can only be properly understood and applied with reference to the function and physiology of the cochlea, so this is where we must begin. To help our understanding, a computer graphics model of the cochlear travelling wave is provided on CD. The history and prehistory of OAEs is then revisited to see how OAEs have evolved to where they are right now. Finally, after briefly introducing OAE technology and practice, I look at the future potential and role of OAEs and highlight some still unanswered questions.

# COCHLEAR FUNCTION:
# THE KEY TO UNDERSTANDING OAES

The cochlea's sole function is to act as an interface between the physical world of sound and the brain and it does this via a neural transmission system that evolved long before wide frequency range hearing organs developed. Birds, reptiles, and amphibia typically only hear up to only a few kiloHertz (KHz) and they achieve this against limits imposed by the slow speed and ill-matched signal transmission characteristics of nerve pathways. Mammalian cochleae have a very effective solution to this problem. It involves the travelling wave mechanism first described by von Bekesy and is illustrated later in this chapter in conjunction with an interactive computer program on the accompanying compact disc.

The travelling wave mechanism gives the mammalian ear an action similar to the eye in that it projects a spatial image of the stimulation it receives onto its sensory epithelium (Figure 1–1). This serves to distribute sound energy comprising a very wide range of sound frequencies across some 3,000 inner hair cells by focusing different frequencies on to different places of the organ of Corti (Figure 1–2). It is important to remember that auditory nerve fibers are *not themselves* frequency specific at all, but depend on the inner hair cells to select their input. Inner hair cells too are more like low-pass filters and respond to whatever the travelling wave delivers. Much depends on the quality of the travelling wave.

In contrast to the lens of the eye, the ear performs its physical role of "image forming" in a counterintuitive way—a kind of mixture of a prism and lens for vibration. Like the eye, the mechanism for the production of this spatial image of frequency components is inherent in the physical characteristics and anatomical construction of the cochlea. But there is no obvious refocusing mechanism in the ear and the physics behind the process is entirely different and an order of magnitude more complex.

There are many functional benefits of the travelling wave mechanism for the ear. First, distribution of sound stimulus energy across cells by frequency relieves individual auditory nerves fibers of having to convey the individual cycles of vibration of the original sound—which they do badly above 500 Hz. Nearly all of the useful information available in a narrow band of frequencies is carried by the fluctuations in amplitude of the waveform. Extraction of this information—a process known as demodulation—is naturally provided at each place in the cochlea by the asymmetrical mechano-electrical nonlinearity (rectifying action) of the inner hair cells (Figure 1–2). High frequency hearing then ceases to be a physiological problem. The auditory nerve is never actually presented with high frequencies—but only with the lower frequency modulation! With this mechanism some aquatic mammals achieve a frequency range of over 12

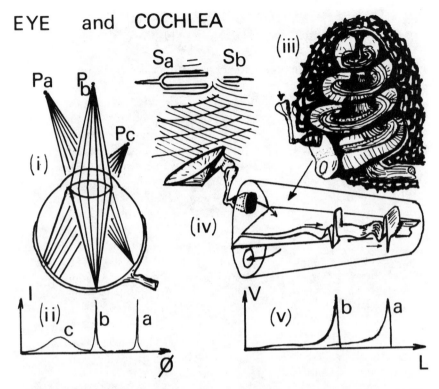

EYE   and   COCHLEA

**Figure 1–1.** Both the eye and ear create a spatial image of the outside world. The direction of light determines the places of energy focus on the retina (ii). The distance and lens setting determines resolution. For the ear the frequency of sound determines the place of focus in the cochlea. The larger tuning fork makes a lower frequency sound, Sa, which is focused nearer to the apex of the cochlea (iii). The higher frequency sound from the smaller fork, Sb, is focused nearer the base. The one dimensional spatial image in the ear is crudely one of the SIZE of the sound radiating object (iv). The sounds of mice and of twigs breaking go to the base, lions roaring and thunder go to the apex! The resolution (v) is critically determined by level of frictional remaining after the outer hairs cells have responded.

octaves. Small rodents are able to achieve the directional hearing they need despite their small interaural distance by working at ultrasonic frequencies.

There are further benefits to the ear if sharp vibration focusing is achieved. The sharper the focus on the organ of Corti, the stronger the peak of excitation achieved for each single frequency, resulting in enhanced detection sensitivity. The sharper the focus, the more strongly is interfering information at other frequencies rejected, resulting in greater noise immunity—greater frequency selectivity. Finally the sharper the focus, the nar-

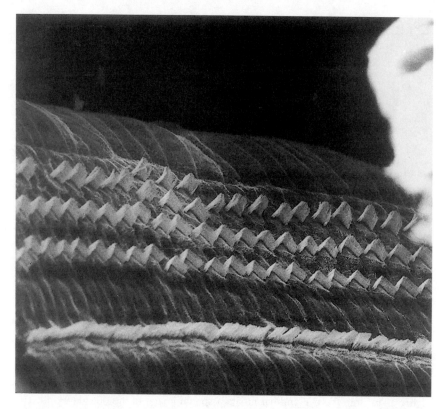

**Figure 1–2.** The surface of the organ of Corti showing the inner hair cell stereocilia (nearest row), which alone drive the auditory nerve and the three rows of outer hair cell stereocilia beyond, which govern organ of Corti motion. The organ of Corti rides the travelling wave as it moves along the basilar membrane. The physical reaction of each outer hair cell nudges the wave along, giving it extra energy and combating the effects of friction. (Electron micrograph of the guinea pig cochlea by Andy Forge, Institute of Laryngology and Otology.)

rower is the bandwidth of frequencies presented to each hair cell, resulting in a reduction in the rate of information flow through each inner hair cell and nerve fiber. The ideal is to have the information bandwidths of all sections of the system—travelling wave, inner hair cell, and auditory nerve—all matched. These principles will be very familiar to today's mobile telephone engineer seeking to compress more telephone calls into limited bandwidth capacity, and all are biologically advantageous, too.

The first step in really understanding and using OAEs is to recognize that the "quality" of the cochlea's mechanical response to sound—the quality of the spatial "image" of sound it achieves—is crucial to normal hearing sensitivity and selectivity.

So if we want to detect and examine sensory hearing loss, and if pathology in *any* way affects this image, then we absolutely must have a means of assessing the quality of the cochlea's physical response to sound. This leaves us with two questions. Does pathology affect the travelling wave? How can we assess the travelling wave and image quality in the cochlea to look for damage?

The travelling wave *is* very easily damaged by pathology, and OAEs are by far the best way to examine this vital cochlear function.

## THE COCHLEAR TRAVELLING WAVE

The physical response of the cochlea to physiological levels of sound stimulus is very difficult to observe. This is not due only to the cochlea's inaccessibility but also to the small scale of motion in the ear. The motion of hair cells is actually subatomic at threshold, and even very loud sounds move the cells less than one stereocilia width! Textbooks (and our computer model) show hugely exaggerated motion.

Sixty years ago von Békèsy painstakingly observed the pattern of basilar membrane vibration. In order to see any motion of the basilar membrane under the microscope, he needed destructively loud sounds—in excess of 120 dB SPL—applied to "deaf" (cadaver) ears. Although he had no conception of the cochlear amplifier and otoacoustic emissions, his description of the cochlea's mechanism for sound separation and focusing is still very much applicable today. As Békèsy first described, and as is shown on the CD program, the pattern of vibration induced by sound on the basilar membrane is a snakelike wave motion travelling along the basilar membrane at speeds 100 to 1,000 times *slower* than sound. This slow wave is initiated by the sound pressure applied to the fluid of the scala vestibuli by stapes motion and consists of the energy transferred from stapes to the basilar membrane during the sound presentation. The details of this wave motion are still the subject of intense mathematical study, but contemporary texts are not always helpful to clinicians and audiologists with neither the time nor mathematical background to fully digest them! However, the general characteristic of the cochlear travelling wave is easy to appreciate and useful in understanding OAEs.

The travelling wave is a dynamic event in the cochlea, poorly represented by static figures. A computer graphics teaching program for PCs is provided on compact disc with this book (Brass & Kemp, 1998). The program is not a quantitative research tool and it comes with apologies to those who have spent their lives developing much more accurate and realistic models! Appendix A in this chapter gives details of the program and how to operate the software.

The demonstration program shows the up and down motion of the (straightened out) basilar membrane greatly magnified and in slow motion. Waves travel from left (base) to right (apex) across the screen, reaching a peak of some sort then rapidly diminishing. The human cochlea is of the order of 30 mm long and spans some 10 octaves. If the population of hair cells was equally divided between these octaves (which it is not quite), then there would be approximately 300 hair cells responsible for processing each octave of sound. Since the resolution or auditory bandwidth of human hearing is approximately one third of an octave it follows that approximately 100 hair cells serve to transcribe the peak of the travelling wave for any one frequency. This is a surprisingly low number. Furthermore, as the waves reach their peak, their speed slows down greatly, and the waves bunch together, as can be understood from the computer model illustration. The peak itself contains a number of wavelengths of vibration. So at the peak, the individual upward and downward components of the travelling wave may each be served by only a handful of inner hair cells!

Figure 1–3 and the initial settings of the computer program illustrate just how two different frequency tones, entering the cochlea simultaneously, travel toward the apical end and are subsequently separated yielding two distinct peaks of excitation. Figure 1–3A depicts both the excitation envelope and a "snapshot" of the travelling waves in response to two equal amplitude continuous tones, one at 6 kHz and the other at 1.5 kHz, sampled after 40 ms of stimulation. The program can be paused and continued at any time by pressing the space bar. Dynamic equilibrium has been reached. The two octaves of frequency separation give a wide spatial separation (several millimeters) of the excitation peaks on the basilar membrane, with the higher frequency terminating first, nearer to the base. In Figure 1–3B, tones of 4 kHz and 2 kHz are presented. The separation distance is less. The lower frequency tone ($f_1$) is clearly of significant amplitude underneath the peak of the higher frequency tone ($f_2$) and would mask the latter if the level of $f_1$ was raised, but as it is, the peak of $f_2$ itself is still distinct.

The cochlear image does not develop instantaneously—and this explains some of the latency of OAEs. Figure 1–3C shows the 4-kHz and 2-kHz tones in 3B, but after only 5 ms. The higher frequency tone's excitation envelope has quickly reached dynamic equilibrium, while the lower tone's envelope is still growing. The peak of excitation grows as energy accumulates. By counting the complete waves under fully developed travelling wave (in the figure about 4 waves) you can easily estimate the latency of initial activity at the place of the peak-to-be as 1 ms at 4 kHz, 2 ms at 2 kHz. The full development of the peak takes longer. If this model cochlea were to generate a backward travelling wave from the peak, there would be a delay of at least 4 ms between entry of a sound and the maximum re-emis-

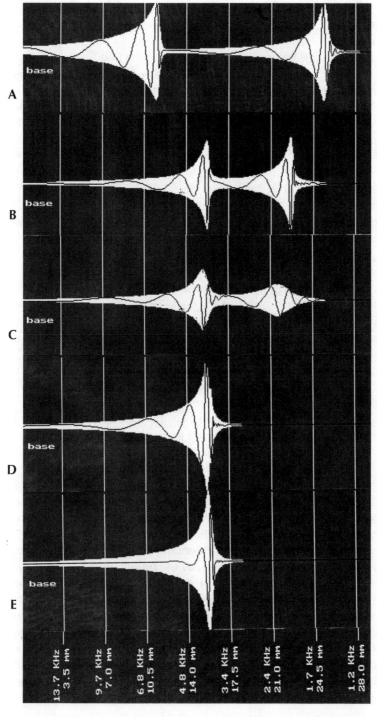

**Figure 1–3.** Travelling wave envelopes generated by the teaching program supplied on CD with this book. **A.** $f_1 = 1.5$ kHz, $f_2 = 6$ kHz, Level $L_1 = L_2 = 2$. Damping parameter 0.4 Screen print at 20 ms. **B.** as A but $f_1 = 2$ kHz, $f_2 = 4$ kHz. **C.** as B but sampled at 5 ms. **D.** $f_1 = 3.9$ kHz, $f_2 = 4$ kHz $f_2/f_1 = 1.03$ Seen in the in-phase state. **E.** as D but in the out-of-phase state. The scale shows the loss free place frequency at interval along the model cochlea.

sion from the cochlea. Actual human OAEs at this frequency have a somewhat longer latency, rodents have less (Kemp & Brown, 1983; O Mahoney & Kemp, 1995).

Neural activity could of course be initiated by the first waves to reach a place—if they were strong enough—so it could be the case that the travelling wave was still developing inside the cochlea (and even being re-emitted as an OAE) after the compound action potential had signaled the arrival of the sound and ended (see also Norton & Neely, 1987).

The limiting resolving power of hearing is set by the travelling wave. Figure 1–3D and E show the response to two tones too close together to be resolved by this cochlear model. Only one peak is seen. The frequencies involved, 4 kHz and 3.9 kHz, have a ratio $f_2/f_1$ of 1.03 and a frequency difference of 100 Hz. Every 1/100 s these tones move in and out of phase with each other resulting in beats (see Figures 1–5 and 1–9). In Figure 1–3D, the tones are in phase and the travelling wave looks "normal." In 3E, the tones are out of phase at the stapes and over much of the basal region of the basilar membrane. The result is apparently no stimulation over the basal region! However, the energy already stored in the travelling wave is still present and is seen highly localized to the peak. This demonstrates how the envelope of the travelling wave depends on the exact form of the stimulus and is itself dynamic. A pair of tones can present a quite different pattern of excitation to a single tone, and this is relevant to DPOAE generation.

The reason for the rise in vibration amplitude of a travelling wave going apical along the basilar membrane is the reduction in wave propagation speed. This is easily seen on the computer model. The primary physical cause is the basilar membrane becoming more compliant and wider with distance. As the travelling wave slows down, the energy it contains is concentrated into a smaller distance and the amplitude of vibration increases (Brass & Kemp, 1995). Wavelength correspondingly decreases, but the vibration *frequency* of course stays the same. (Count the waves N passing a mark on the computer screen each second, and the distance $\lambda$ between peaks near to the mark to find the screen velocity $\lambda/N$.) As a consequence of the increased amplitude of vibration there are higher velocities of transverse (up and down) motion. Membrane motion means motion passed fluid and hence viscous drag. So, as the travelling wave develops apically along the basilar membrane, it slows down, concentrating the energy in a higher amplitude of vibration and leading to increased energy loss. At some point along the route the rate of loss of energy by friction in each section becomes equal to the gain in energy in each section due to the concentrating action. This point defines the peak of the travelling wave where it ceases to grow. Dissipation of energy rapidly accelerates after that point as the wave slows down more and it dies very quickly. The greater the viscous drag within the cochlea, the shorter distance the wave is able to travel before it ceases to grow and begins to decay, that is, increased damping moves the reduced travelling wave peak basally.

In a notionally lossless cochlea, the travelling wave would continue to grow until it reached a point at which its velocity was zero and its amplitude of vibration infinite. This point would be analogous to a place of resonance in a simpler system. In practice it is never reached, as there is always damping. The wave and other waves of higher frequency cannot travel apically from this point and vibrations of equal or higher frequency imposed on the basilar membrane apical to this point cannot travel basal apically or basally. This is relevant to the differential propagation of DP components (see below).

In the real cochlea the important thing to note about the travelling wave is that the smaller the viscous damping, the sharper and higher will be the peak achieved by the travelling wave. Damping within the cochlea therefore determines the peak intensity of the excitation delivered by a particular sound and to a lesser extent, the place of the peak along the basilar membrane. In general cochlear damping becomes relatively greater when high stimulation is applied. (In the model the damping increase will have to be applied manually.)

It has already been noted that the full resolution of the cochlea takes time to develop. In Figure 1–4A, continuous tones of 4 kHz and 3 kHz ($f_2/f_1$ = 1.33) are observed in the cochlea after just 3 ms. These frequencies are of a ratio sometimes used for DPOAE measurement. There is no clear separation of the frequencies at this early time, only one broad peak. After 20 ms (Figure 1–4B) full frequency separation is obtained. This process of wave buildup and frequency separation can be prevented by damping— taking away energy faster than it can accumulate. In Figure 1–4C, the damping (energy loss) in the cochlea has been increased by 4 times and the same stimuli applied. Even after 20 ms, the two frequencies are not well resolved. The travelling wave envelope is also smaller by 3 times. The owner of such a cochlea would suffer a threshold elevation of 10 dB and discrimination loss as a result. In Figure 1–4D, the damping is increased ten fold. The travelling wave gets smaller still and there is only one broad peak. In an ear the threshold elevation would be 18 dB and the tones of 3 kHz and 4 kHz would not be resolved at all.

Figure 1–4 presents a good model of sensory hearing loss due to outer hair cell dysfunction. External amplification can restore the amplitude of the travelling wave—but not the separation of frequencies. In Figure 1–4E, a 20-dB increase in stimulus input amplitude is seen to produce a larger but single broad peak at the place normally the focus of 4.8-kHz tones. An inflexion in the travelling waveform is all that identifies $f_2$ as being present. There is always a basal shift of maximum excitation if damping is increased. The loss of resolution also means that low frequency tones can

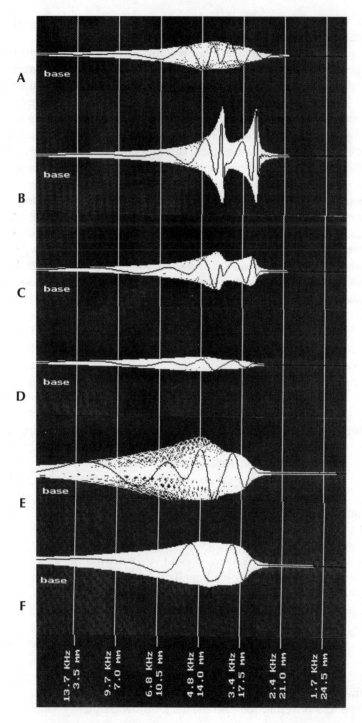

**Figure 1–4.** Loss of resolution cannot be compensated for by amplification. **A.** as Figure 1–3 with $f_1 = 3$ kHz and $f_2 = 4$ kHz sampled at 3 ms. The travelling wave peaks have not yet developed. **B.** as A after 20 ms, showing fully developed peaks **C.** as B but with 3 times more damping present. **D.** as B but with 10 times more damping present. **E.** as D but with stimulation increased by 10 times. **F.** as E but with $L_2$ reduced by 10 dB.

more easily mask higher frequency tones. In Figure 1–4F, the level of $f_2$ is decreased 10 dB. All traces of the $f_2$ stimulus go.

It is a remarkable feature of the cochlear imaging system that the image it forms of a pure tone of any frequency is essentially the same shape! Look at Figure 1–3A. The more apical peak (1.5 kHz) is vibrating 4 times more slowly than the basal peak (6 kHz). The wavelength and shapes are almost identical—just shifted. The perceptual mechanism can therefore "recognize" that this is a pure tone—whatever its frequency—by the neural image of the travelling wave envelope shape. Real life sounds are rarely pure tones, but contain a wide range of frequencies. The range of frequency which can be effectively radiated by a sound source is actually determined by the shape and size of the source. One need only think of the deep sounds made by large objects and animals, and the thin sound made by small creatures. Here we come nearer to the truth about what the cochlea is really built to do. It places different sounds within a spatial image of the sound environment according to the *size and scale* of the sound source—a feature of obvious advantage for survival (see Figure 1–1 text).

## DISTORTIONS OF THE TRAVELLING WAVE—THE SOURCE OF OAEs

The cochlear travelling wave determines the quality of sound reception. We have seen how its shape depends on the stimulation, how the peaks representing individual frequencies take time to develop, and how they become depressed if damping is increased. All this comes from the teaching of von Bekesy. Simple linear passive versions of the cochlea, which he envisaged, will not re-emit the sound it receives—it all gets absorbed sooner or later. This changes if the travelling wave becomes distorted.

Distortion exists in various forms in the cochlea—deviations from the "ideal" physical structure, distortions to the smooth gradation of stiffness and mass along the basilar membrane, irregularities in hair cell properties and arrangement, mechanical nonlinearity in the displacement of stereocilia. These all lead to distortions in the *envelope* and phase progression of the travelling wave and/or to the *waveform* of the vibration it carries.

The phenomenon of otoacoustic emission requires only that some significant part of the cochlea's forward travelling wave energy gets turned back—reflected or scattered. The travelling wave describes the flow of energy in the cochlea. Distortions to the travelling wave are distortions to the energy flow. If the travelling wave hit a brick wall it certainly would reflect energy back to the middle ear (look ahead to Figure 1–15B), but would a minor disarrangement of hair cells, or a dead or overactive hair cell, initiate a returned wave? How about mechanically nonlinear motion of the stereocilia—if they resisted motion more on the up than the down wave—what would that do? What are the necessary conditions for some travelling wave energy to be returned?

Supported by the first observations of otoacoustic emissions (Kemp, 1978c) it was hypothesized that in the real, healthy cochlea the travelling wave *is* reflected to some extent by the action of the sensory cells. To quote from that paper:

> *Retrograde energy transfer in the cochlea can occur only in special circumstances. as observed by Bekesy in model studies (Bekesy 1960) viz. the source of excitation must be on the basilar membrane and extend over a region of mechanical imped-ance gradient. It is hypothesised here that impedance discontinuities arise in the cochlea because of a mechanical response of the transduction mechanism to stim-ulation leading to a travelling wave reflection. (p. 1386)*

In other words, otoacoustic emissions were from the outset considered to be echoes of a distorted travelling wave. This proposition was strongly resisted by the auditory research community, despite the strong experi-mental evidence presented. The OAE response waveform to a click showed the same order of delay and frequency dispersive behavior as might be expected from the return of a high quality travelling wave. There was clear evidence of nonlinearity (distortion) in the click-evoked response with changing stimulus level (Kemp, 1978c), and distortion products them-selves were recordable as otoacoustic emissions (Kemp, 1979a). The issue was debated at the First International Symposium on Active on Nonlinear Mechanical Processes in the Cochlea held at the ILO in 1979 and published in full in *Hearing Research*, Volume 2, 1980.

There was a polarization of opinion. Evans neatly summarized the concerns of many at the 1979 London meeting:

> *I think many of us now would be happy with the conclusion that these echoes, whatever they are have an intracochlear origin. However there has been resistance to this conclusion on a number of grounds. . . . One is the long latency of the echo which seems to me to be too long to explain in terms of basilar membrane stand-ing waves or whatever, if people believe that any more. And the second question is how exactly is this energy propagated out of the cochlea? That's a problem many of us found very difficult, particularly when the reflection was accounted for in terms of basilar membrane mechanics. (Evans from Kim, 1980a)*

In support of the concept of returned travelling waves, Hall (1975, 1980) had already published computations of bidirectional propagation along the basilar membrane and Kim, Siegel, and Molnar (1977) had already analyzed the relationship between basilar membrane nonlinearity and distortion product propagation. However, neither of these groups had considered including the middle ear in the computation in a way which would include sound radiation from the ear. After the presentation of distortion products from the human ear at the Inner Ear Biology Workshop in Seefeld in 1978, Kim was the first to realize this omission and went on to be the first to extend the observation of DPOAEs to laboratory animals (Kim, 1980b).

The question of how and why the cochlea travelling wave returns some of its energy to form otoacoustic emissions occupied the minds of leading auditory theorists (e.g., de Boer, 1980). The matter is still not fully resolved. Nevertheless, distorted echoes of the travelling wave do emerge.

## UNDERSTANDING DPOAES

Distortions to auditory perception, as opposed to distortions of the travelling wave, have been widely recognized for hundreds of years. Tartini wrote about it in 1714 and Helmholtz in 1856. A large body of psychoacoustic literature this century has documented the properties of the "intermodulation distortion" heard between two pure tones.

Despite the existence of aural combinations tones, few believed that they implied mechanical distortion affecting basilar membrane vibration until the advent of DPOAEs. In support of the "linear cochlea" view was evidence that combinations tones were heard clearly even at quite low levels which necessitated a quite unusual form of nonlinearity—not of the "overloading" type (Goldstein, 1967). Even the "overloading" type of nonlinearity was absent from pre-1978 recordings of basilar membrane motion at moderate levels of stimulation with the exception of Rhode (1971) who reported nonlinear vibration in squirrel monkey cochlea. At high levels, overload nonlinearity occurs in the middle ear and cochlea. Dallos was first to observe and discuss the distortion created by overloading effects in the ear by means of ear canal acoustic recordings (Dallos, 1966, 1973), although these were very different from DPOAEs. But for the most part, during the 1970s, cochlear mechanical nonlinearity was considered to be irrelevant to normal cochlear function.

The advent of DPOAEs permitted aural combination to moderate level tones to be objectively recorded for the first time. The basic DPOAE technique is simple. The ear canal is closed by the probe to retain the sound created by tympanic vibration. The two pure sound sources must be independent and unable to react on each other. The frequencies are made close enough for the travelling wave peaks on the basilar membrane to overlap. The ear canal sound collected by the probe microphone is narrow-band filtered to select one of the distortion tones created by nonlinear interactions in the cochlea.

Distortion products are not in themselves biological phenomena. Just as harmonics are generated whenever the waveform of a pure tone deviates from a sine wave, so distortion products are introduced whenever the waveform of complex sound—be it a two tone pair, click, or any other sound—is immediately distorted by the effect it has on the system it is travelling through. It happens in hearing aids, hi-fi systems, loudspeakers, and also in ears. The mathematics of distortion is common to all cases and in an appendix to this book, Kevin Knuth provides an excellent tutorial on the subject.

For the nonmathematician, a graphical exposition of how distortions to complex waveforms arise and are translated into new frequency components is provided in Figure 1–5. The figure deals with two- and three-tone signals passing through a system with various degrees of saturating non-linearity. It could represent the signal arriving at the inner hair cells or the signal in an auditory nerve or the output of a hearing aid—or the signal ejected by the cochlea as a backward travelling wave leading to an OAE.

What makes distortion products (and stimulus frequency emissions) from the ear clinically interesting is the wealth of evidence that they reflect the properties of a nonlinear process associated with outer hair cell motility. For clinical purposes, the level of the DP emission "$2f_1 - f_2$" is typically measured for a number of stimulus frequency pairs, covering the hearing range. Many have been tempted to present such DPOAE measurements as a means of objective audiometry. This is incorrect because DPOAEs are generated prior to the excitation of the inner hair cells and of the auditory nerve where threshold is set. However, as "distorted echoes" of the travelling wave, it is reasonable to expect the intensity of DPOAEs to correlate with the intensity of signal arriving at the inner hair cell—and consequently with auditory threshold.

A correlation between auditory threshold and DPOAE level does exist, but it is quite weak due to the many intervening variables which affect otoacoustic emission and not hearing. As a consequence, the prediction of an *individual's* threshold of hearing with OAEs is not possible to any useful degree of accuracy (Kimberley et al., 1997), other than to say whether it is likely to be inside or outside of normal limits. Attempts to define a threshold of DPOAE detection are thwarted by the fact that DPOAEs do not have a physiological threshold, but simply become masked by the instrumentation and patient's (uncertain) noise.

Another misconception is that DPOAEs are a "different phenomenon" to stimulus frequency OAEs and transient evoked OAEs. In fact, both are part of the same complex process. Note from Figure 1–5 that the input tones $f_1$ and $f_2$ survive the nonlinearity and emerge accompanied by distortion products which can be at a comparable level—depending on the nonlinearity. A nonlinear system will in general transmit the input signal and add to it distortion product components.

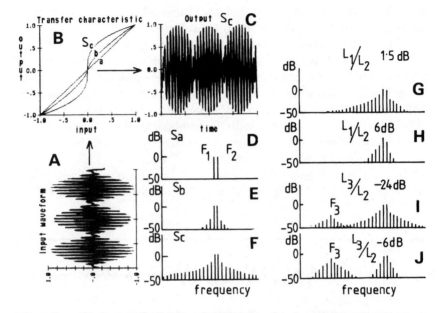

**Figure 1–5.** Distortion product generation and suppression is not in itself a physiological phenomenon. The rules are simple. **A.** Two continuous pure tones have a "beating" waveform. As they pass through a system **B.** the waveform can be distorted if the transfer function is not linear (Sa). The system Sc has a saturating nonlinearity and compresses the higher parts of the waveform. **C.** Distortions to the waveform create new frequency components. The undistorted signal passing through system Sa has only two frequency components $f_1$ and $f_2$. **D.** The response of system Sb introduces intermodulation distortion products, the strongest being $2f_1-f_2$ and $2f_2-f_1$. **E.** The more severe nonlinearity of system Sc generates very many intermodulation products. **F.** The ratio of levels is important. $L_1 > L_2$ produces more lower frequency distortions than upper **G.** and **H.** When a third tone is introduced, new distortion is created of the form $f_3+(f_2-f_1)$ and $f_3$ minus $(f_2-f_1)$ even for quite small $L_3$ (**I**). When $L_3$ is made stronger **J.**, the original distortions around $f_1$ and $f_2$ are reduced. This is suppression. (See corresponding biological data in Figures 1–9 and 1–11.)

If, for example, Figure 1–5E represented the signal returned by the cochlea to the middle ear (i.e., an OAE) then the $f_1$ and $f_2$ spectrum lines would be the *stimulus frequency* OAEs and the other lines would be the DPOAEs. At the middle ear, the emerging OAE signal would meet the (stronger) incoming signal. The stimuli $f_1$ and $f_2$ would overlay the weaker emerging stimulus frequency OAEs at $f_1$ and $f_2$, making them extremely difficult to identify. But the distortion product components would be more easily observable by frequency analysis. If instead of tones, a wide band signal were to be applied, distortion would still occur but now stimulus, stimulus frequency OAEs, and DPOAEs, would all coalesce—as in TEOAEs.

It is always necessary to separate the stimulus and response in OAE measurement, and this is done by exploiting some property possessed by the OAE and not the stimulus. With TEOAEs, it is the inherent delay of the OAE. In DPOAEs, it is the frequency separation. With stimulus frequency emissions, it is the nonlinearity with the stimulus level that is used. Figure 1–6 gives an example of how stimulus frequency and DPOAEs can be extracted with a tone pair combination. Contrary to some accounts, DPOAEs are not instantaneously produced. The stimulus frequency and DP components actually emerge with a similar latency to each other and

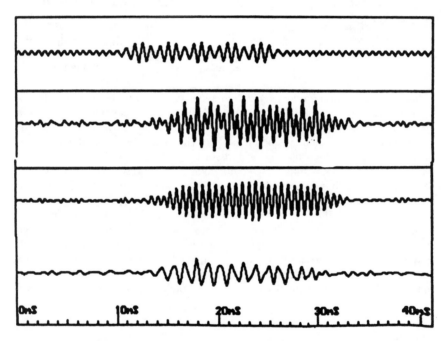

**Figure 1–6.** SFOAEs and DPOAEs are both part of the delayed echo of the travelling wave. A specially constructed two tone complex was used by Kemp, Brass, and Souter (1990) to extract stimulus and distortion product emissions during two tone stimulation. $f_1$ = 1200 Hz, $f_2$ = 1550 Hz, $L_1$ = 70 dB SPL, and $L_2$ = 60 dB SPL. The top trace is a section of the stimulus containing two control periods with $f_2$ only, and a two-tone period. The beat between $f_1$ and $f_2$ at a rate of 1500–1200 is clearly seen as a beat at intervals of 1/300 s. The second trace down is the ear canal signal with all linearly behaving components removed, i.e., only the emission. It is complex and delayed by around 5 ms. From this signal a stimulus frequency OAE at $f_2$, the third trace down, and a DPOAE at $2f_1$–$f_2$ lower trace, can be extracted by filtering. Both have identical delays. Both are part of the "whole OAE."

also have a similar latency to that of transiently evoked OAEs. All stimulated OAEs are delayed OAEs. However, DPOAE latency is a particularly complex parameter (O Mahoney & Kemp, 1995; Moulin & Kemp, 1996) and must be carefully quantified according to the method of measurement as illustrated in Figure 1–7. This is because DPOAEs depend on two inputs $f_1$ and $f_2$, each of which have a different latency.

To understand a little more about how DPOAEs arise and how they should be interpreted we need to look at the travelling wave again. Figure 1–8 shows distortion products on the model basilar membrane. In Figure 1–8A, the travelling waves and excitation envelope during stimulation with equal amplitude tones of 4 kHz and 3 kHz $f_2/f_1 = 1.33$ are shown. It is often repeated that DPOAE comes from the "geometric mean frequency

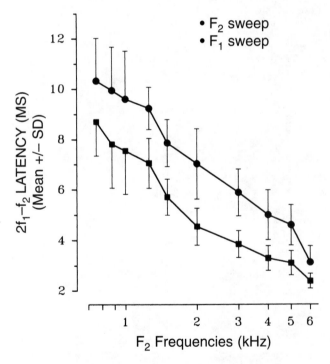

**Figure 1–7.** The latency of the DPOAE $2f_1–f_2$ in human ears as a function of frequency. It is close to that of TEOAEs but does not have a singular value. Here it is estimated by phase gradients during incremental sweeps of either the $f_1$ or $f_2$ tones. $L_1 = -65$ dB SPL, $L_2 = 60$ dB SPL, $f_2/f_1 = 1.2$. $F_1$ sweeps give lower latency than $f_2$ sweeps. Standard deviation bars indicate substantial differences among the 12 adult subjects. (From " Multicomponent Acoustic Distortion Product Otoacoustic Emission Phase in Humans II. Implications for Distortion Product Otoacoustic Emission Generation, by A. Moulin and D. T. Kemp, 1996. *Journal of the Acoustic Society of America, 49,* pp. 1640–1642. Reprinted with permission.)

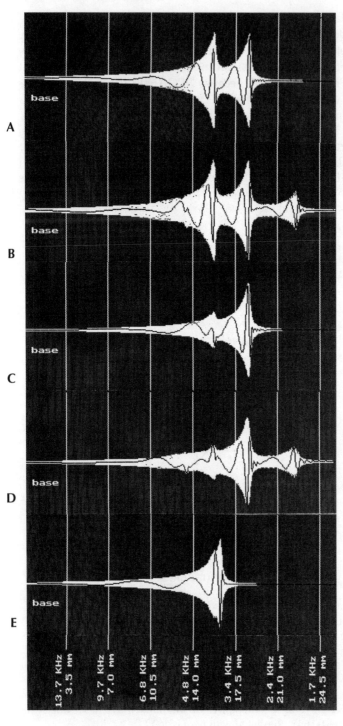

**Figure 1–8.** A travelling wave view of distortion products. In **A.** tones of 3 kHz and 4 kHz are imaged by the model cochlea as in Figures 1–3 and 1–4. In **B.** nonlinearity is added and leads to the production of $2f_1-f_2$ and $2f_2-f_1$. The former travels to its own place on the basilar membrane, apical to the $f^1$ place. $2f_2-f_1$ is of higher frequency than $f_2$ and this gives rise to maximum vibration basal to the $f_2$ peak—at its own place. **C.** The level of $f^2$ is dropped by 12 dB SPL in the linear condition so that the levels of $f_1$ and $f_2$ are more similar where they interact. With nonlinearity reintroduced the $2f_2-f_1$ is now more clearly seen in the travelling wave **D.** In **E.** the stimulus frequency ratio is reduced to 1.03 and the two tones are not separately resolved by the cochlea. The travelling waves overlap as do those of $2f_1-f_2$ and $2f_2-f_1$. For close primaries the generation of both DPs and their re-emission probably happens at the same place.

place" which lies midway between the two peaks. It is hard to trace the origin of this idea but Figure 1–8A shows this place to be in a region where the 4-kHz tone ($f_2$) does not even reach. DPOAE cannot be generated there except for very close primary frequencies. Equally clear is the fact that, from the base to the peak of the $f_2$ wave, both $f_1$ and $f_2$ are present as a vibration of the basilar membrane—and so they *could* interact nonlinearly to produce a distortion at any place along it. Wherever they interacted along the cochlea, the DPOAE *frequency* would be exactly the same frequency, $2f_1$–$f_2$. The DP frequency does not tell you where the OAE was generated.

In Figure 1–8B, a general nonlinearity is added to the model to create distortions. The intermodulation distortion product $2f_1$–$f_2$ is seen travelling past $f_1$ peak to its own place apical to the $f_1$ peak—just as in Kim's experiments (1980b). The DP wave could have been produced over a large portion of the basal cochlea where $f_1$ and $f_2$ coexist—there is no way to tell just by measuring the DP.

We have already seen from Figure 1–5 that distortion products are not solitary tones but come in sets. The companion to the widely studied distortion product $2f_1$–$f_2$ is $2f_2$–$f_1$ and it is of a higher frequency than $f_2$. Because it is a higher frequency it cannot travel even as far as the $f_2$ place. In the simulation Figure 1–8B, its presence is seen only as an inflexion of the travelling wave at the cochlear peak place of $2f_2$–$f_1$—a point that is at a slightly shorter distance basal to the $f_2$ place as the $f_1$ place is apical. In Figure 1–8C and D, the level of $f_2$ is reduced relative to that of $f_1$, and with nonlinearity (Figure 1–8D) the place of the DP $2f_2$–$f_1$ is more clearly seen.

Figures 1–8B and 1–8D serve to address another fallacy in popular ideas about DPOAEs. It is that the use of *pure* tones, with precisely defined frequencies, to evoke DPOAEs (as opposed to click stimuli) somehow serve to target one highly localized part of the cochlea. The point has already been made that $2f_1$–$f_2$ DPOAE *generation* could occur anywhere from the base of the cochlea up to the peak of $f_2$. Precisely where it occurs depends partly on the ratio of intensities of the primaries at the nonlinearity as illustrated in Figure 1–5.

In common nonlinear systems, total DP production is greatest if there is equality of the two input signals. The intensity ratio at each point on the cochlea depends on both the intensity and frequency ratio of the two primaries. Figure 1–8 helps to explain why. In Figure 1–8A, $f_1$ and $f_2$ are of equal intensity at the input, but the level of $f_1$ is much smaller than that of $f_2$ at the peak of $f_2$. When $L_2$ is dropped by 12 dB the levels of $f_1$ and $f_2$ become comparable at the $f_2$ peak as seen in Figure 1–8C and maximum DP production might be expected at the $f_2$ place. With $L_2 = L_1$ maximum DP production might spread basally where levels of $f_1$ and $f_2$ are more equal. If $f_2$ and $f_1$ come close in frequency the optimum level difference between the two will approach 0 dB as in Figure 1–8E and we would expect most

DP to be generated at the mutual peak. These qualitative arguments are no substitute for precise calculation, but it is clear there is no basis for thinking two tone stimulation automatically pinpoints one very narrow region or even a single cell, as implied by Welch Allyn (1995).

The situation is made even more complex because the *generation* of distortion and the *creation of reverse travelling wave* (and hence a DPOAE) are not one and the same thing. These events may occur at differing places. Furthermore, generation may occur over a wide area, and reverse wave creation may occur at more than one location. During a clinical DPOAE measurement, for example, the DP signal may be generated near to the $f_2$ peak and also be re-emitted from that point to be joined by a DP signal taking the longer route via the DPOAE travelling wave place. The summation of DP components from different locations could be additive or substractive depending on the frequency and ratio of the primaries.

We must therefore regard the relation between DPOAEs (and any other OAE) and the health of individual places in the cochlea to be at best an empirically demonstrated relationship and not a logical necessity. Certainly the precision of frequency specification does not translate into precise place specificity. Models such as Figure 1–8 at least help to provide a basis for deciding what is happening in the cochlea when stimulus intensity and frequency ratio options available on DPOAE instruments are used.

However, Figure 1–8E suggests that there is one condition where we might assume that the generation and emission of DP comes from the peak of primary excitation. It is when $f_2/f_1$ is near 1 and $L_2 = L_1$. Will this condition take us closer to the underlying nonlinear properties of the organ of Corti at one frequency-specific place?

Figures 1–3E and 1–8E illustrate the travelling wave envelopes for this special condition. Figure 1–9 shows the complete anatomy of a close primary DPOAE with experimental data from a gerbil. The levels (60 dB SPL) are quite strong for a gerbil and a wide range of DP frequencies are produced. Reference to Figure 1–5D, E, and F shows that this is typical of strong and sharp (high order) nonlinearities. In the model (Figure 1–5F), however, equal numbers of DPs appear above and below the primaries. In ears the upper range is always restricted. This difference between model and experiment actually helps to confirm that most of the DP generation is happening at the primary peaks, from which frequencies above $f_2$ cannot escape from the cochlea (see above). By filtering out the energy at the stimulus frequencies, we can recreate the "whole" DP waveform (Figure 1–9 lower trace). It's not a sine wave—it contains many nonharmonic components which add up to a series of sharp tonebursts. Each burst represents the reaction of the cochlear nonlinearity to one cycle of the beating effect in the stimulus waveform (center trace (a) in Figure 1–9)—each one a miniature TEOAE!

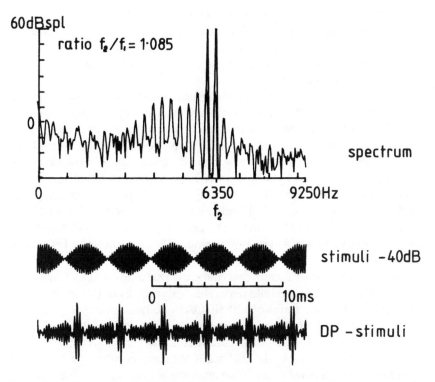

**Figure 1–9.** The anatomy of DPOAEs. Top spectrum of ear canal sound pressure in a gerbil during stimulation with tone tones at $f_2$ = 6350 Hz and $f_1$ = 5852 Hz ($f_2/f_1$ = 1.085) $L_1$ = $L_2$ = 60 dB SPL. Many DPOAEs are under these conditions, from $9f_1$–$8f_2$ below $f_1$ to $3f_2$–$2f_1$ above $f_2$ (see Kemp & Brown, 1986). Center, the stimulus waveform reduce by 40 dB showing the beats between the primary tones. Bottom, the actual waveform of the complete DP complex, showing the sound bursts echoing the reaction of the cochlea nonlinearity to the beats in the stimulus. This trace was obtained by subtracting the stimulus frequencies from the ear canal signal. Synchronous averaging was applied to enhance signal to noise.

## OAE FREQUENCY SPECIFICITY—WHAT DOES IT MEAN?

Frequency specificity is generally regarded as a "good thing" in an auditory response, but the term is used in a number of different ways. It is commonly used to imply that a tonal stimulus evokes a response relevant to the hearing of that frequency. A logical extension of this is that the response comes from the anatomical region responsible for processing that frequency—this is *place specificity*. OAEs have the additional characteristic, shared with the cochlear microphonic response, that they are *synchronous* with the stimulus. This means the response is at the same frequency as or *locked to* the stimulus frequency. The compound action potential has this property only weakly at low frequencies, and the ABR does not have this feature. But CAP and ABR do have frequency place specificity. The cochlear microphonic is a strongly synchronous response but has very poor frequency place specificity.

OAEs therefore are unique in being *synchronous* and to some extent *frequency place* specific. This unique property means that, even when presented with a wide band click stimulus, each part of the cochlea can give an OAE response at its own place-specific frequency. The resulting multifrequency specific information can be carried simultaneously by a complex OAE and *then* decoded by frequency analysis to give multiband frequency (place) specific data. That's how TEOAE analysis works. In contrast, if the ABR is measured using click stimuli, all frequency specificity is lost. With OAEs it is not. So TEOAEs and DPOAEs are potentially both highly frequency specific. Welch Allyn (1995) completely misrepresents TEOAEs in this respect.

A number of other factors determine the usefulness of OAE frequency specificity. First is the threshold dependence dynamic range. CAP and ABR have a wide dynamic range of 120 dB. OAEs do not, having only 30 dB or so. This limits OAEs to frequency-specific screening. The second factor is the correlation between response parameters and threshold elevation. The absolute amplitudes of both ABR and OAEs are poorly correlated with threshold. They depend strongly on anatomical and skin conductivity factors. However, ABR detection threshold is well correlated with the audiolmetric threshold, but OAE detection threshold is not. Accurate threshold predictions can be made with ABR but not with OAE.

The third factor to consider is resolution (i.e., how small and well defined a region of the cochlea can we obtain information about). This depends on the source of OAE within the travelling wave—and as we have seen for DPOAEs this is not always very well defined. There is no reason to believe that TEOAE resolution is any better or worse.

The best empirical source of evidence as to the cochlear place being "tested" during a DPOAE or TEOAE measurement is suppression tuning curves (e.g., Figures 1–10 and 1–12). To obtain a DP tuning curve a third tone is introduced and varied in level and frequency to determine the combinations that suppress the DP by a predetermined amount. For a fixed criterion, such as 6 dB of DPOAE suppression, a V-shaped tuning curve is obtained, as in Figure 1–10 for $2f_1-f_2$. High frequency slopes are always steep, corresponding to the abrupt termination of travelling waves in the apical direction. The low frequency slope is always less. The latter corresponds to the rise of the travelling wave (Brass & Kemp, 1993). A range of low frequency slopes are found for different individuals and for different stimulus combinations. The frequency of maximum ease of suppression is

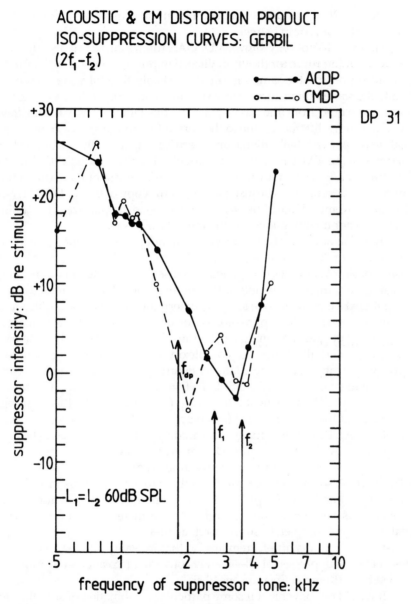

ACOUSTIC & CM DISTORTION PRODUCT
ISO-SUPPRESSION CURVES: GERBIL
$(2f_1-f_2)$

**Figure 1–10.** DPOAE and CM DP have similar origins. Suppression tuning curves of $2f_1-f_2$ distortion product in a gerbil. Tone stimuli $f_2$ was 3600 Hz, $f_1$ 2700 Hz. $L_1 = L_2 = 60$ dB SPL. Both the ear canal sound and the round window cochlear microphonic contain distortion products with similar tuning curves. (From "Ear Canal Acoustic and Round Window Correlates of $f_1-f_2$ Distortion Generated in the Cochlea," by D. Kemp and A.M. Brown, 1984. *Hearing Research, 13*, pp. 39–46. Reprinted with permission.)

rarely at the $2f_1-f_2$ frequency. Depending on the primary levels and ratios, it can be at $f_1$ or $f_2$ or in between.

Figure 1–10 not only shows a DPOAE tuning curve but also the suppression tuning curve for the $2f_1-f_2$ distortion present in the cochlear microphonic response to the same stimuli. Remarkably, the CM also shows practically the same tuning curve. How should we interpret this? Does the CM distortion come from the same place as the DPOAE? We would have expected some differences due to the very different transmission and summation properties of vibrational and electrical signals in the cochlea. Alternatively, is the CM DP, actually the regular basally produced CM to the DPOAE vibration as it returns to the base—as a new stimulus? The tuning curve of CM would then be just a microphonic copy of that of DPOAE (see Brown & Kemp, 1985). The example serves to emphasize that tuning curves do not unambiguously settle the "place" issue.

The idea of using of a third tone as an independent pointer to explore the "place" or "reception frequency" relevant to a DPOAE signal is in any case too simplistic. DPOAE generation itself is complex enough—how much more complex is the interaction of three tones? If we cannot assume that DPOAEs come from one logically determined place in the cochlea how can we assume that the suppression action of the third tone ($f_3$) acts at a logical place? Suppression tuning curves must be interpreted with caution.

Figure 1–11 illustrates the complexity of three tone DP generation, already indicated by model data in Figure 1–5I and J. A human ear's response to primaries at 70 dB SPL, $f_2/f_1 = 1.211$ and $f_2 = 2734$ Hz, shows the expected DP components $2f_1-f_2$, $3f_1-f_2$, and $2f_2-f_1$. In this example, when a third tone $f_3$ of 1599 Hz (just below $2f_1-f_2$) is introduced, also at 70 dB SPL, the DP $2f_1-f_2$ is actually enhanced by 3 dB while $3f_1-2f_2$ is heavily suppressed. At least five more DPs appear including $2f_3-f_1$ and $2f_2-f_3$, which are the cubic distortions between alternative pairs of primaries—$f_3$&$f_1$, $f_3$&$f_2$. Also a totally new family of three-tone DP appears including $f_3$ minus $(f_2-f_1)$ and $f_3 + (f_2-f_1)$! This family is more clearly shown in Figure 1–5I and J as a cluster of lines around $f_3$. As $f_3$ is increased in level, the original $2f_1-f_2$ gets completely suppressed, as predicted. The new family $f_3 + n(f_2-f_1)$ and $f_3$ minus $n(f_2-f_1)$ remains, so that in reality DPOAE generation has not been suppressed at all—merely converted into another form—controlled by $f_3$ (Kemp & Sivanessan, 1998).

It would be convenient if some particular combination of stimulus led to a simplification of DP production. A useful simplification is afforded by widening the primary separation and turning to the upper DP $2f_2-f_1$. Figure 1–12 is for primaries at 70 dB SPL with $f_2/f_1 = 1.4$. The DP $2f_2-f_1$ must now be generated at place well basal to the $f_2$ place, well away from the peaks of $f_1$ and $f_2$, and in a region where $f_1$ and $f_2$ vibration are uniformly equal over a wide region. The lack of stimulus gradients will mean that no additional frequency dependence of the action of $f_3$ on the DP will be

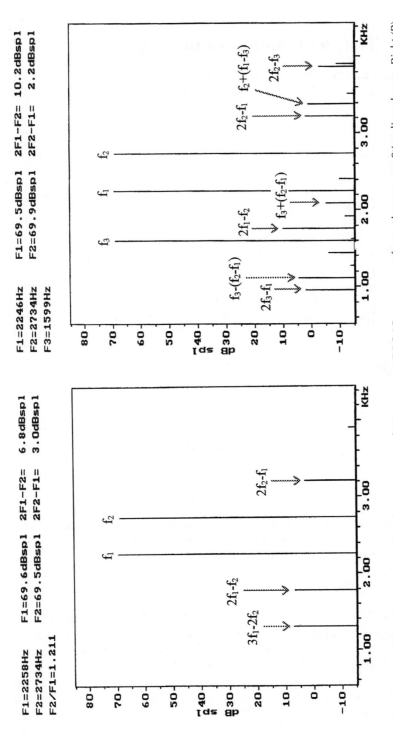

**Figure 1–11.** DPOAEs are a complex phenomenon. Left (A) common DPOAE component from a human ear. Stimuli as shown. Right (B), introduction of a third tone results in new DPs, frequencies as marked and discussed in the text. Tuning curves for DPOAEs derived by means of a third suppress seldom take into account the complexity of the process.

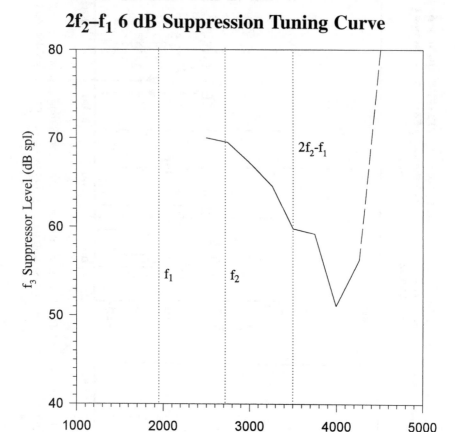

## $2f_2-f_1$ 6 dB Suppression Tuning Curve

**Figure 1–12.** Paradoxical DPOAE tuning curves. A human suppression tuning curve of the DPOAE $2f_2-f_1$ for $L_1 = L_2 = 70$ dB SPL $f_1 = 2700$ Hz $f_1 = 1950$ Hz. The curve shows a maximum susceptibility 1/5 octave above the DP frequency for 6 dB of suppression. Suppressors around $f_1$ and $f_2$ barely affect $2f_2-f_1$ DPOAE generation. (Data collected by S. Sivanesan using the three-tone ILO96)

imposed. Also the potential for DP generation will be uniform. Only the predisposition to transmit a DPOAE will be tested when $f_3$ is swept in frequency. The result is an interesting tuning curve where the peak of suppression occurs with $f_3$ set 1/5 octave above the suppressed DP.

If we take a simplistic view of the experiment in Figure 1–12, we would have to conclude that, when all other things are equal and there are no nearby primary peaks, then DPOAE production is most susceptible at a place somewhat basal to the peak place for the DP frequency. Regular $2f_1-f_2$ production also broadly peaks when $f_2$ is 1/4 to 1/3 octave above $f_1$ (ratios $f_2/f_1$ 1.8 to 1.26), i.e., when the $f_2$ travelling wave peak sits on the rising slopes of the $f_1$ peak. The frequency range of DP products also seems to have fixed frequency limits around $f_2$ (Kemp & Brown, 1986). Brown and Williams (1993) proposed a secondary mechanical filter to explain these phenomena. Some believe that the basal slope of the travelling wave is the most effective site for "cochlea" amplification.

OAEs have been described as the result of distortion to of the "natural" form of the travelling wave. This distortion seems to begin in a region somewhat basal to the travelling wave peak, at a place where energy input is possibly taking place and nonlinearity most prominent. Nonlinearity energy input and position are therefore all major factors in OAE production. Determining the health of outer hair cells in this "special" region would seem to be the aim of any frequency-specific OAE test.

This brings us back to the need for power assistance for the cochlea, which we first introduced to compensate for the effects of damping in the cochlea and to enhance the focusing of travelling waves to differing frequencies. Amplification is certainly one of the most remarkable properties of the cochlea. We now trace the origin of this concept to the eventual identification of OAEs.

## AN HISTORICAL DIVERSION

Science seldom progresses in a straight line—and sometimes doubles back on itself. Such has been the case with our understanding of the cochlea's response to sound. Auditory biophysics and physiology took an unproductive detour beginning in the late 1940s which possibly delayed the discovery of hair cell motility and of otoacoustic emissions by 40 years. It is worth examining the reasons for the detour.

Helmholtz anticipated the importance of having a good frequency selective cochlear response to vibration in the mid 19th century. He could not directly observe it, nor did he know of the physiological necessity for it. Rather his ideas were based on intuitive reasoning and parallels between musical instruments and the anatomy of the cochlea. The mid 20th century saw von Bekesy greatly develop this concept with his revolutionary travelling wave theory. Originally a telephone research engineer, Békèsy belonged to the pre-electronic era. He accepted, without question, the poor resolution of the sound focusing mechanism that he found within dead cochleae as a reasonable consequence of the natural viscous drag of the fluid in the narrow spaces of the organ of Corti. It indicated to him, and most other auditory physiologists before 1980, that the ear must be depending on some other "higher" mechanism for its resolving power.

Pathology—even death—would surely have little effect on the physics of his travelling wave!

Thomas Gold, on the other hand, was experienced in radio and electronic engineering and was working on hearing in the physiology laboratory in Cambridge, England, at that time. Gold knew that the sensitivity of a radio receiver could be ruined by excessive loading of the antenna. He also knew that the signal response characteristics of any system—including the degree of damping—could be altered by means of an "active element" and by "feedback." The transistor had just been invented in 1948, but the active element available to electronic engineers at the time was the thermionic vacuum tube or "valve." Electronic feedback had also been widely used to improve radio receiver characteristics prior to the introduction of superhetrodyne (frequency shifting) technology (see Figure 1–13).

From his experience with radios, Gold felt sure that the cochlea must contain the biological equivalent of the vacuum tube, as he related: *"Surely—nature can't be as stupid as that—to put a nerve fibre—that is a detector—right at the front end of the sensitivity of the system"* (Gold, 1989). As to the possible mechanism for response enhancement, he saw the cochlear "microphonic" potential as playing a vital role in the process together with the reverse (electrical to vibrational) process by which it appeared to be possible to "hear" the frequency of a large oscillatory electric field applied (dangerously) near to the ear.

In his 1948 paper, he writes prophetically:

> *Let us assume . . . that the cochlear microphonic effect results from a modulation of a further source of energy as could be supplied by some form of electrochemical action.* [now recognized as the function of stria vascularis] *The acoustic energy which would be required to modulate an electric current could theoretically be arbitrarily small.* [now recognized as the energy to work the outer hair cell ion channels]. *We then see that with this one assumption . . . about the nature of the cochlear microphonic effect we have a feedback channel. An oscillating fibre of the basilar membrane would produce an electric field. This would in turn by means of the second (electric to mechanical ) transducer* [now identified as the outer hair cell "motor"] *result in a mechanical force impressed on the fibre. . .*

He continued by spelling out exactly what this meant—and was absolutely right:

> *We would then regard the cochlea as no longer a passive instrument where nerve endings merely record the displacement due to an applied force, but as an active mechanism where an applied signal releases a chain of events involving an additional supply of energy. . . . First and most importantly of course the feedback action may largely cancel the resistive losses and would thereby enable* [basilar membrane] *fibres to oscillate as a "high Q element." . . . The locus for this action*

*might be . . . the hairlets spanning the gap between Corti's arches and the tectorial membrane. . . . If the feedback ever exceeded the losses then a resonant element would become self oscillatory, and oscillations build up to a level where linearity was not preserved. A permanent adjustment of* [sufficient] *accuracy would seem to be impossible when we consider the unsteadiness of the framework, and some form of self regulating device would have to exist* [now attributed to the efferent system].

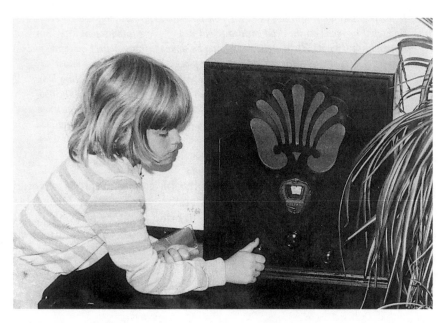

**Figure 1–13.** Early radio receivers (wireless sets) made use of positive feedback (regeneration) to compensate for resistive losses in the tuning circuits and antenna. The technique was invented by Armstrong in 1913 and patented (the Audion, USA patent No. 1113149) and the improvement it brought to reception precipitated the introduction of "broadcasting." Amplified radio signals were injected back to the coil, which selected the radio station. Performance could be very good, with high sensitivity and selectivity, but instability was a problem. Frequent adjustment of the feedback was needed as the set warmed up and aged. If wrongly set, oscillation would occur, distorting the radio station with a whistle, and emitting radio waves via the antenna into the ether—causing a whistle on neighboring listeners' sets! The positive feedback method soon became old technology when in 1919 Armstrong invented an even better method—the "superhetrodyne" technique (not yet thought to be present in the ear). But the positive feedback method was simpler, cheaper to implement, and persisted in low priced radio sets until well into the 1920s and 1930s as illustrated here. Gold was well aware of the strengths and weaknesses of technique and adopted it as a model for the cochlea action in 1948. The cochlea, however, seems to have overcome most of the disadvantages of the method.

It is interesting that Gold wanted high quality (high Q) low-loss oscillatory responses in the cochlea. This was primarily to explain psychophysical measurements of the frequency discrimination characteristic of the ear which he made with the physiologist R. J. Pumphrey (Gold & Pumphrey, 1948). At this time, of course, Bekesy was still developing his travelling wave theory based on direct cochlear observation—in cadaver—and was reporting very low quality (low pass filtering) responses. Gold later recalled:

> I had discussed at length in 1948 with von Bekesy at Harvard, that the observations that he made on the dead cochlea [Gold, 1989], were unrepresentative. But he wouldn't have it! He thought there must be some cunning neural mechanism that somehow steepens up the subjective response. But Bekesy also I must say seemed quite unaware of the necessity to apply the correct physical scaling laws between the large models he built and the observations on the cochlea that he had. . . . So I returned from my meeting with Bekesy even more convinced that I was correct. . . . before I met him I had the view point that maybe these great men had something up their sleeve that we don't know about. . . . but I became more convinced that we really had to pursue this [theory].

Consider how differently auditory physiology and biophysics would have developed if these two men had understood each other and been able to work together. Bekesy was well placed to bring auditory physiology out of the 19th century. But Gold was already well into the 20th century and ahead of his time. He was the first to propose hair cell motility, the cochlear amplifier, and the adjusting mechanism we now attribute to the cochlear efferent system a generation too early. He was also even on the brink of discovering OAEs as the following quotation shows.

> In spite of such a self regulating mechanism we might expect that occasional disturbances would bring an element into the region of self oscillation. If this occurred then we should hear a clear note . . . until the adjusting mechanism had regained control. . . . If the ringing was due to actual mechanical oscillation in the ear then we should expect a certain fraction of the acoustic energy to be radiated out. A sensitive instrument may be able to pick up these oscillations and so prove their mechanical origin. This would be almost certain proof of this theory. . . .
> Gold actually searched for these sound emissions by placing one of the microphones of the day near to an ear. When we attempted this we did not succeed in making our ears ring with the required persistence. Further . . . the sound energy available outside [the ear] would only barely exceed the noise level of a sensitive amplifier (Gold, 1948).

Gold had predicted spontaneous otoacoustic emissions as a consequence of misadjustment of the amplifier mechanism. Despite the instrumentation limitations of his day, Gold probably could have detected true

SOAEs if he had looked for *continuous* pure tones in the sealed ear canal of healthy young ears, as Glanville et al. (1971) unwittingly did some years later—but he did not. We know today that the commonly experienced spontaneous loud fading "ring" type of tinnitus Gold sought to measure is probably not of the SOAE type.

Gold's preoccupation with "ringing" came from his belief that there needed to be high Q resonances in the cochlea. To explain frequency difference limens around 0.1%, he and Pumphrey had proposed auditory filter bandwidths of less than 1/230 octave compared to the 1/3 octave we accept today! Pumphrey and Gold were wrong on this point. The physical basis of frequency discrimination is not the narrowness of the auditory filter but its sharp high frequency limit with a slope of over 500 dB/octave. The lateral translation of this very sharply apical termination of the travelling wave envelope required only a frequency change of 1/500 octave in a pure tone to bring a detectable 1 dB change in excitation to the few hair cells occupying the position of the sharp termination.

But at the time, Gold had no reason to doubt the high Q filter hypothesis and he systematically explored its consequences. It required loss reduction in the cochlea (therefore an active process) and indicated a long ringing time for elements in the cochlea. All filters ring with a time constant inversely proportional to their bandwidth ($Tc = 1/[\pi\text{bandwidth}]$). So a simple 1-kHz filter with a Q of 300 (bandwidth 1000/300 = 3.3Hz) would have a ringing time constant of around 50 ms. Gold knew this was a very long time to propose for the ear and had to answer strong criticism on this point. He recalled:

> This prompted people to object that ringing after a stimulus would take such a long time that it would have been readily observed in previous measurements. I kept having to explain that the Q of an individual fibre does not determine the length of time for which the oscillation could be heard outside the ear. . . . Rather it was the unevenness of the frequency coverage that the cochlea provided that specified . . . the duration of the ringing after a stimulus. However no one at that time really did any sensitive experiments of this nature and the argument—that it would already have been observed—was just used against my theory (Gold, 1998, p. personal communication)

When defending his cochlear amplifier/high Q resonator theory Gold apparently had to argue against others' suggestions of delayed *stimulated* otoacoustic emissions—or at least ringing—from a healthy uniform ear! His counter-argument was that self-cancellation of the responses from different parts of the basilar membrane to the same stimulus would prevent the internal workings of the cochlea from ever being observed in the ear canal—unless there was disorder. Bekesy would have agreed with Gold on this point. His travelling wave theory emphasized that wave propagation along the basilar membrane was always from base to apex. So, if any oscillation was generated inside the cochlea—it could simply not escape to the middle ear. Without supporting evidence, Gold's theory was effectively excluded from further consideration. Psychophysicists disagreed with the need for high Q resonances, Bekesy disagreed with the need for an active cochlea, and everyone agreed that sound could not escape from the healthy ear!

Although initially spurred on by Békèsy's rejection of his hypotheses, Gold was eventually finally beaten back by the apparent ignorance he encountered among the otologist and neurologist that he tried to enthuse with his ideas: "I got very discouraged and instead I invented theories of cosmology and one thing and another, and drifted out of the hearing field" (Gold, 1989 p. 301). Gold went on to have a very distinguished career in cosmology and geophysics but he still maintains an active interest in hearing science.

## SHARP RESONANCES RE-EMERGE!

Paradoxically in 1958, high Q sharp resonances in human hearing were actually reported by psychologist Elliot (1958) (see Figure 1–14). His work on standards for audiometric threshold at the British National Physical Laboratory revealed sharp peaks and dips in audiogram—about 50 Hz wide between 1 and 2 kHz (Q = 40). Van den Brink (1970) and Thomas (1975) also reported narrowly defined undulations in the pitch of sounds and in the threshold of hearing, respectively. As with Gold's work, these papers aroused little interest at the time.

My own psychophysical research revealed that the threshold peaks and valleys were associated with various other anomalies found in normal hearing including loudness enhancement peaks and aural distortion. Detailed mapping showed what appeared to be sharp physical resonances within the auditory system (Q>50) associated with an "active" mechanism. The original 1976 abstract (Kemp & Martin, 1976) is reproduced here as an appendix to this chapter (Appendix B).

What really interested me was finding a rational explanation, not of hearing itself, but of the bizarre findings and also the sheer novelty of a complex mechanism precisely definable by psychophysical measurements (Figure 1–15A). Although the experiments were performed through headphones in a sound booth, it was like examining the response of a defective hi-fi system in a large reverberant room. A pure tone near to threshold would at one frequency be clear, but 50 Hz higher would be inaudible. At one frequency it would seem to be pure—at another to be rapidly pulsating or double. On switching off the tone at a frequency giving a slowly beating effect, an internal tone might persist at the same frequency, then fade. In some extensive but clearly mappable domains of frequency and amplitude, diplacusis occurred which could be attributed to intermodulation of the stimulus tone with an inaudible internal tone ($f_2$) causing $2f_1-f_2$ to be heard. Related effects had previously been reported by Wegel (1931), Flottorp (1953), and Ward (1955), but again no one had interpreted the phenomenon as being of relevance to cochlear function.

The previous experience I had with radio propagation research proved invaluable. I had studied the way sub-audiofrequency radio waves from thunderstorms echoed many times around the world exciting specific resonances of the whole earth ionosphere cavity (fundamental frequency 8 Hz) (Kemp, 1970). The "Q" of these resonances (4–6) depends on the electrical resistance of the ionosphere which in turn depends on the solar wind. One of Gold's major achievements after leaving auditory physiology was to explain the behavior of the solar wind at the magnetosphere. For me entering auditory physiology as an applied physicist, my experience with geophysical responses made a number of things about the auditory

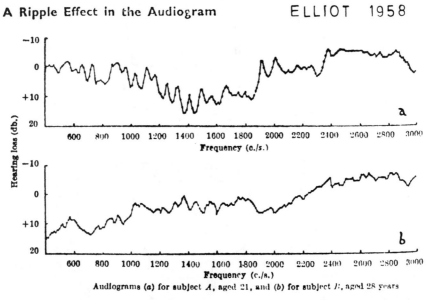

Figure 1–14. Detailed (15-Hz interval) audiometric threshold measurement in two subjects showing sharp changes in threshold, up to 10 dB over 30 Hz. This means that standards for clinical threshold determination have to allow a ±5 dB margin for the hit or miss effect and that threshold may appear to vary—when in fact it is the audiometer frequency which has changed slightly! It is now accepted that these peaks are the effect of multiple internal reflection of otoacoustic emissions. (From by . Elliot, 1958, p. Nature, 181, p. 1076. Reprinted with permission.)

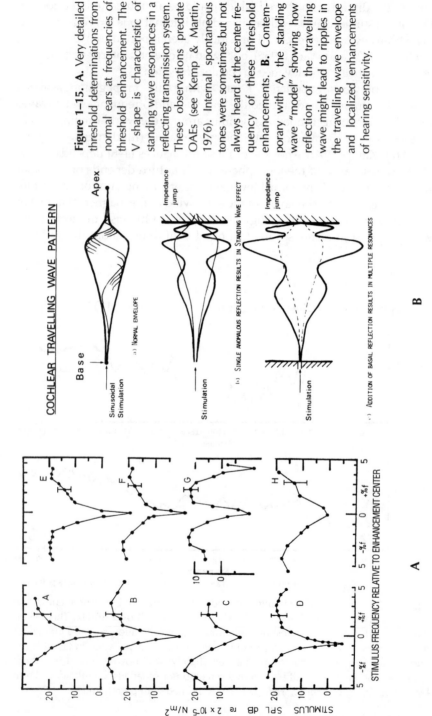

**Figure 1–15. A.** Very detailed threshold determinations from normal ears at frequencies of threshold enhancement. The V shape is characteristic of standing wave resonances in a reflecting transmission system. These observations predate OAEs (see Kemp & Martin, 1976). Internal spontaneous tones were sometimes but not always heard at the center frequency of these threshold enhancements. **B.** Contemporary with A, the standing wave "model" showing how reflection of the travelling wave might lead to ripples in the travelling wave envelope and localized enhancements of hearing sensitivity.

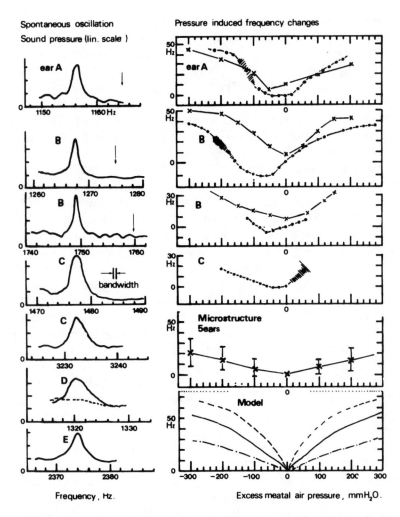

**Figure 1–16.** Left, a study of seven spontaneous sound emissions from different subject with normal hearing. The bandwidth of the analysis was 0.16 Hz. Each SOAE sampled over 1 min has a bandwidth of 1–2 Hz, so each is not a pure tone. Allen, and also Bialek and Wit (1984), have fiercely debated if the broadening is due to wandering of a pure tone or is evidence that SOAEs are simply highly filtered thermal noise. Right, the behavior of four of these emissions under tympanic displacement invoked by positive and negative ear canal pressure. The U-shaped changes in frequency show that the stiffness of the tympanum plays a role in frequency determination, as model studies show (bottom panel). The same evidence can be obtained by observing changes in the threshold enhancement frequencies (second panel up) (From Kemp, 1981). Spontaneous OAES are not therefore due to one place in the cochlea going into oscialltion—but to a large part of the cochlea osillating with the middle ear—driven by one overactive place.

microstructure come together to provide a model—if not an explanation—for Elliot's threshold peaks and valleys.

First, the microstructure phenomenon was peripheral not central as Elliot has supposed, because middle ear manipulation altered the frequencies of microstructure effects (Figure 1–16, right). Second, it was vibratory in nature because beats could be heard with external tones. Gold had proposed such a test of internal cochlear oscillation (Gold, 1948). Third, it was a nonlinear phenomenon because the loudness peaks and valleys levelled out at higher sound levels—and because $2f_1-f_2$ aural distortions interacted with the phenomena (Figure 1–17A). Finally, and crucially, it was a systematic phenomenon—the loudness peaks and threshold minima tended to be uniformly spaced in frequency at around 100 Hz between 1 and 2 kHz (Kemp, 1979b). Systematic peaks and valleys in loudness and threshold could be accounted for if the cochlea reflected the travelling wave back—to cause standing waves and a regular interference pattern (Figure 1–15B). If the round trip results in minimal energy loss, then multiple internal reflections between middle ear and active cochlear region are possible—but only for frequencies that have whole number of cycles per trip. High Q resonance would then be the result of constructive interference and multiple internal reflections at suitable frequencies. The interresonance interval in such a system is the reciprocal of the round trip delay.

Békèsy had clearly demonstrated that the travelling wave was heavily damped, but the auditory microstructure phenomenon showed this to be untrue for the healthy human ear. This in turn made it necessary to propose amplification to reduce the impact of damping and allow the sound energy to reflect backwards and forward along the cochlea at threshold—and this amplifier would explain the remainder of the phenomenon. Gold had deduced the need for an active mechanism in the cochlea on intuitive grounds and to support a new theory of hearing. I needed amplification to make sense of a strange psychophysical phenomenon. Both reasons involved high Q resonances—but for quite different reasons. Both of us were familiar with the early design of radio receivers involving feedback and both of us understood its potential for amplification—and oscillation. But, as in Gold's day, it seemed to me that no one in the audiological field was ready and able to debate the significance of these findings. *Nature* declined my paper on the auditory microstructure in 1976. Some of this psychoacoustic work was later published in support of OAEs (Kemp, 1979B).

## ENGINEERING A "NEW" AUDITORY RESPONSE

The sequence of events that led to the delineation of OAEs began with psychophysical observations in 1975 and culminated in a series of acoustic experiments beginning in August 1977. In an adjacent laboratory, physi-

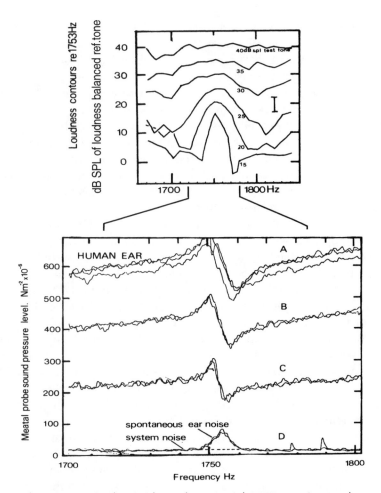

**Figure 1–17.** Further evidence from crucial 1977 experiments that the microstructure of the audiogram is associated with effects on tympanic impedance. **A.** The top panel shows equal loudness contours across a narrow loudness enhancement centerd at 1760 Hz for several stimulus levels from 10 to 40 dB SPL. An alternate tone balancing technique was used against a tone of the same level but kept at 1 kHz in the same ear. **B.** In the lower traces A, B, and C show ear canal sound pressure measurements during stimulus frequency sweeps at fixed loudspeaker drive voltage set to give mean sound levels of 21, 26, and 31 dB SPL. Inflexions of the ear canal sound pressure obtained occur exactly at the peak of the loudness enhancement. The stimulus oscillator and narrow band hetrodyne analyzer were locked together. When the analyzer was swept across the frequency range, this time without stimulation—a spontaneous peak in noise was found at 1754 Hz—the frequency of a tonal tinnitus. The spontaneous emission itself seemed non essential—it was not always present but the other features shown were.

cists John Knight and Chris Green were searching for objective tinnitus with a 1-inch B&K microphone. Without even sealing the microphone to the ear canal, they had recorded some palatal clicks. I reasoned that the vibrations which I knew must be inside the cochlea would also move the tympanum so they must be causing some measurable sound vibration. I knew that the internal cochlear reflection reached the middle ear because tensioning the eardrum with pressure predictably shifted the frequencies of threshold and loudness maxima and minima (Figure 1–16, lower right, and Figure 1–17A) and also changed the frequency of the associated tonal tinnitus. Although this model contradicted contemporary dogma about cochlear travelling waves, it seemed worth trying to measure acoustic correlates of the auditory microstructure.

A precision microphone was not needed so I sealed a miniature hearing aid microphone over the opening of my ear canal. The microphone was connected to a tunable hetrodyne analyzer with a square bandwidth of 10 Hz and an 80-dB noise rejection figure. I found that I could manually tune into my 1764-Hz "tinnitus" at around 10 dB SPL (Figure 1–17D) and found other tones with the probe in other ears (Figure 1–16, left). When I applied a tone of 40 dB SPL at 2 kHz to my ear via an external headphone a new sound was both audible and detectable at 1518 Hz: the $2f_1-f_2$ distortion product between the 1764-Hz internal vibration and the applied 2-kHz tone. Finally, when two external tones were presented at about 60 dB SPL, the $2f_1-f_2$ distortion product was strong enough to be detected in real time when the tones were close (1/2 octave) and when the $2f_1-f_2$ frequency fell near to an enhancement peak of the audiogram.

Figure 1–18 is from this series of experiments and documents the first ever objective recording of the $2f_1-f_2$ DPOAE in August 1977. These experiments proved the physical basis for the microstructure phenomenon and proved the existence of an active nonlinear energy source in the cochlea— to me at least. Interestingly, there remains controversy about what is adequate proof of the cochlear amplifier (e.g., Allen & Fahey, 1992)—and some experiments continue to model the interaction between spontaneous emissions and external sounds to study the amplification process (Tubis & Talmadge, 1998).

My first experiments did not prove the cochlear reflection hypothesis (see Figure 1–15). To go further and prove that standing waves were occurring in the cochlea, the sound level in the ear canal was recorded during a slow sweep of frequency with constant stimulator drive voltage. The input of any system that contains standing waves must show impedance maxima and minima with frequency. This should have and did happen in the ear. Tympanic impedance was affected by the cochlea—but only when very low stimulus levels were used. The subjective peaks and valleys in threshold and loudness were mirrored by undulations in the closed ear canal

## Cubic difference tone acquisition

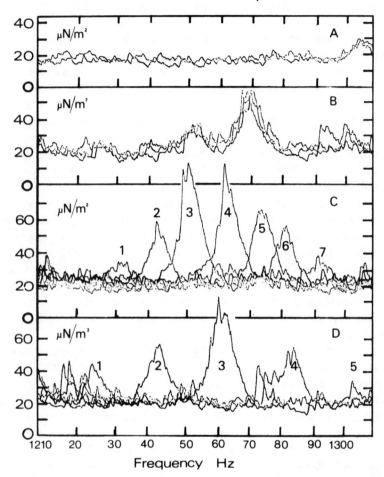

**Figure 1–18.** The first documented objective recordings of the DPOAE $2f_1-f_2$ obtained with a mechanically scanned hetrodyne analyzer with bandwidth 10 Hz in 1977. **A.** The noise level, inside a 1-cc cavity. **B.** The noise across the band with the probe in my ear without stimulation. Spontaneous oscillation is observed around 1260 Hz, the peak frequency of a resonance in that ear. **C.** Analysis of sound developed in the ear canal with a stimulus of 1500 Hz at 60 dB SPL plus a second at 1767, 1758, 1748, 1738, 1727, 1720, or 1709 Hz labeled 1 through 7, always at 60 dB SPL. In each case the $2f_1-f_2$ distortion component is visible. This did not happen in the cavity. **D.** As above but with a fixed 1738-Hz stimulus and the second tone at 1480, 1490, 1500, 1510, or 1520 Hz, against 60 dB SPL. The $2f_1-f_2$ component to each pair is again visible. (From Kemp, 1979b.)

sound pressure (see Figure 1–17, lower part, also Kemp, 1997b, for the original data). The inter-peak frequency gave the round trip delay time of around 8 ms.

All of these phenomena were observable only with near-threshold stimulation. The cochlea was certainly behaving as a loss-free transmission line but only at low stimulus levels. The observations did not seem to me to be a problem for theories of hearing at moderate levels. My problem was how and where to publish a series of physical and psychophysical observations that appeared to others to be at variance with auditory theory and appeared to me to be understandable only to an acoustics engineer!

It seemed at first a trivial extrapolation to demonstrate the phenomena in the time domain—with a click stimulus and an averager rather than a swept tone and a narrow band analyzer (see Figure 1–19A and also Kemp and Sivanessan, 1998, for original data). Obviously, the returned wave from the cochlea would show as a series of echoes, with the delay already determined from the frequency interval between threshold minima—around 10 ms—just as I had seen the electric field from giant lightning strikes echo around the earth. The first experiments on my ear, and of Chris Green's and Trish Lewis's ears, worked (Figure 1–19B). What was unexpected was the complexity and individuality of the echo received from different ears. A whole new technology of TEOAE analysis has evolved to deal with this (see Figure 1–20).

Hallowell Davis visited the department that summer and gave an introductory talk on auditory responses (all electrical at that time). This suggested a new way of presenting the phenomenon for publication. Seen as a stimulus-response sequence the phenomenon would be immediately meaningful to clinical audiologists in a way that distortion products and tympanic impedance fluctuations were not! An echo waveform, well separated in time from the stimulus, was clearly a "response" from the ear—not "magic with signals." A new cochlear response had been invented—the "evoked cochlear mechanical response" or ECMR as it was first called. The publication plan initially failed. *Nature* rejected the paper announcing "delayed sound emission from the ear" in December of 1977 on the grounds that the phenomenon was of specialized interest only. The referee's comments reveal how reasonable and apparently fair criticism can stifle the publication of new unexplained observations:

> *The phenomenon described by Dr. Kemp is most interesting and perplexing and the experiments appeared to be carried out most carefully. However, it is a phenomenon of specialised interest with no obvious explanation. We would suggest that the paper is published in a specialised journal e.g.* Acta Otolaryngology, *where it will attract suitable attention from other clinicians. If in future Dr. Kemp is able to repeat these observations on experimental animals rather than human*

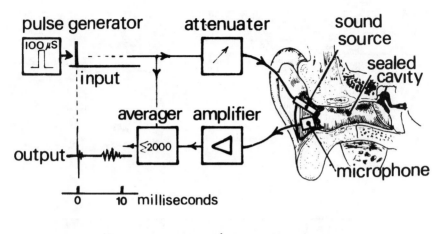

A

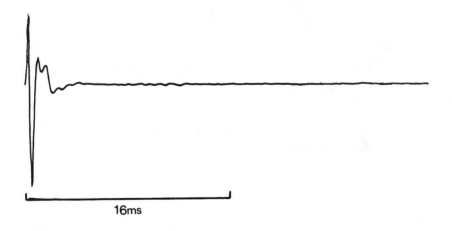

B

**Figure 1–19.** Transient evoked OAEs. **A.** A schematic of the experimental system. **B.** A complete ear canal waveform trace after averaging, showing the input click followed by the oscillation of the ear canal and tympanum, and finally after around 6 ms the signal re-emitted by the cochlea.

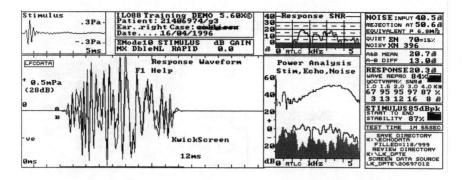

A

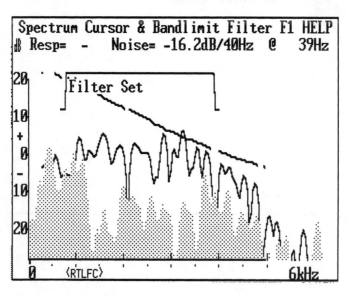

B

**Figure 1–20.** Various ways to analyze OAEs. **A.** The typical transient evoked recording from a healthy infant showing stimulus and response waveforms, signal-to-noise ratio across frequency, and a comparative power analysis with frequency of the stimulus, OAE response and noise. Test conditions and OAE data summary are tabulated right. The test took 115 seconds using the ILO88DP. **B.** An expanded frequency analysis on a linear frequency scale **(B)** shows spectral detail with many fine notches and peaks. The phase plot (line sloping from top left to bottom right) in contrast is remarkably smooth. Its gradient reveals the latency of OAEs by frequency. **C.** To remove unnecessary detail and provide data at audiometric frequencies a half octave power analysis is useful. Finally, in **D.** a comparison is made with DPOAE collected using the same machine and probe. It took 120 seconds. In this example, DPOAE is marginally stronger than TEOAE. This can be reversed in other ears. The DPOAE has a dip at 2 kHz, not present in the TEOAE. As the DPOAEs are

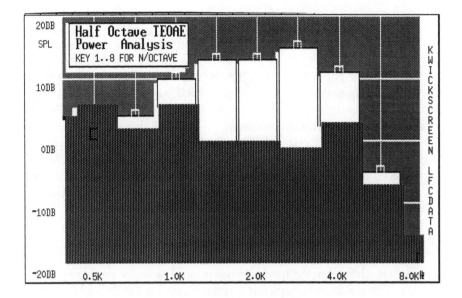

C

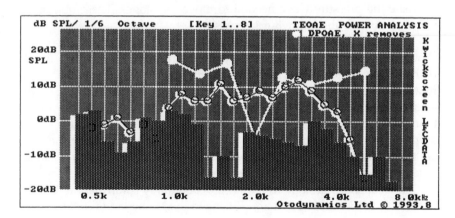

D

complex responses and are collected at spot frequencies, individual points are not always representative of a frequency range. The TEOAE method provides an unbiased panorama of activity but equally can have strong features with no audiometric correlates. TEOAEs usually can obtain a response to lower frequency stimuli than can the DP method. However, TEOAEs often fail to acquire OAEs above 5 kHz in many adult ears whereas DPOAEs succeed. In conclusion, a TEOAE plus DPOAE combination measurement is recommended for clinical investigations. (Example recorded by L. Kimm.)

*patients, and to discover the underlying mechanisms, then this work may be suitable for publication in* Nature. *As it stands the observation is interesting and unexplained, but possibly of potential use in the diagnosis of hearing disorders.*

Contrary to the referee's recommendation, Gold of course had found the otological fraternity of his day to have little use for such physical observations! It is also curious that data from animals would have qualified for publication whereas data from humans was considered suspect!

The first public presentation of OAEs was at the British Society of Audiology meeting at Keele University in April 1978 (Kemp, 1978b also reproduced in Appendix C to this chapter). Here more informed criticisms of the "cochlear echoes" centered around two important issues. The first was how to eliminate the possibility that the sound was created by muscular reflex activity in the middle ear. This was eliminated by showing the absence of adaptation with high stimulation rates. The second objection to OAEs concerned the cochlear travelling wave. There was great reliance on Bekesy's teaching that the traveling wave could never be made to travel in reverse. There was also suspicion that the latency of OAEs could not arise within the normal process of hearing, and that even if a reverse travelling wave was created, it would reach the basal end of the cochlear quite unable to create the pressure wave needed to move the stapes. These objections faded away over the following 10 years.

Strangely, back in 1948, Gold also argued that the healthy cochlea should not reveal its internal response to stimulation. When told of the cochlear echo phenomenon in 1978, he found it hard to believe and later he recalled: *"I must admit I was too negative on that—that one could evoke a stimulated emission. . . . If the* [responses of] *neighbouring fibres* [of the basilar membrane] *were neatly overlapping as they should be to make a smooth curve then you would get practically nothing out* (Gold, 1989). *"I certainly did not appreciate that my theory had any medical applications, but I only thought of experiments that would help to prove it"* (Gold 1998, personal communication).

Otoacoustic emissions were first independently confirmed by Wilson in the U.K. (1980) and by Wit and Ritsma in the Netherlands (1980).

## THE (SLOW) RISE OF OAE TECHNOLOGY

The potential application of the new auditory response was clear from the outset. OAEs could be used to objectively detect sensory hearing impairment with an acoustic probe—and no electrodes. So why did it take 20 years for OAEs to become routine? It seemed at first that it would take only a few months, so we set out to prepare the ground! The averager we used to make the first OAE measurements was a heavy primitive unit previous-

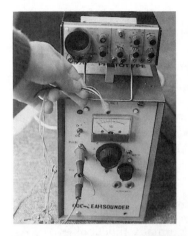
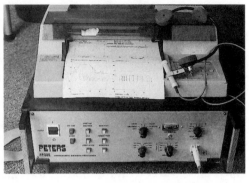
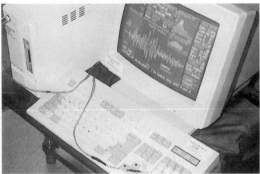
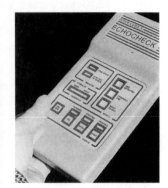

**Figure 1–21.** Four generations of OAE instruments. Top left, the 1978 Cochlear Sounder, a battery portable TEOAE system with nonlinear stimulation, analog averager, and CRT waveform display constructed by R. Chum at the RNTNE Hospital London. Top right, the 1985 Peters AP200 microprocessor-controlled TEOAE system with nonlinear stimulation, artifact rejection, stimulus and response frequency analysis, and plotter display. The first commercial OAE system manufactured by A. Peters Sheffield U.K. and based on specifications developed at the ILO, University College London. Bottom left, the 1991 version of the ILO88 personal computer based OAE system built by Peter Bray of the ILO. It featured color VDU real time FFT displays and online monitoring of all parameters. Screening, laboratory, and spontaneous OAE modes. Programmable with full data recall—expand. Some versions could record both TEOAE and DPOAE. Forerunner of the ECHOPORT, which was widely used for screening. Bottom right, the 1998 version of the Echocheck pocket-sized, battery-powered, hand-held, DSP controlled TEOAE system developed by David Brass of the ILO. Optimized for screening its features, automatic stimulus evaluation, and response scoring.

ly employed in cortical response research. We needed something to take into the clinic to collect data and to demonstrate to manufacturers. In late 1977, Rudolph Chum and I began to design and build a portable TEOAE instrument in order to demonstrate the method and prove its use in screening. This device we called the "Cochlear Sounder" is shown and described in Figure 1–21A.

A patent had to be filed to protect the investment of any commercial manufacturer interested in developing the device commercially and to help raise funds for further research into OAEs (Kemp, 1978a). It included all devices that comprised an acoustic probe to apply sound to the ear canal and to record the sound in the ear canal, and which additionally used some form of signal processing designed to separate the stimulus sound from the newly discovered sounds returned from the cochlea: sounds that we claimed would indicate a normally functioning cochlea and middle ear. This formal patent claim encompasses DPOAE and TEOAE systems equally.

Audiology depends on the audiological instrument industry and the industry depends on audiologists. The rapid translation of new discoveries and concepts into instrumentation is vital to the health of both. In 1978, we had hoped to see the industry rapidly take over OAEs. Our plan failed. Most manufacturers were in fact formally offered licenses to develop OAEs at various times from 1978 to 1990 including Madsen, Nicolet, GSI, Biologic, and Virtual. Some never replied, some disputed the patent, and some had other plans. There were no takers.

At first, in the early 1980s, there was no real understanding of the importance of OAEs within the audiological instrument industry. By the late 1980s, there was some understanding, of OAES, but a lack of confidence in their potential and a lack of willingness to invest in a new technology or certainly to fund pure research. By the early 1990s (when commercial prospects looked better), there was suddenly commercial activity to develop OAE instruments, accompanied by a denial (at least in the USA) that the DPOAE method came within the scope of OAE master patent! As a result, the Institution which hosted the discovery of OAEs, has so far failed to gain any research funding from the sale of U.S. manufactured OAE systems. It has been argued, by those same manufactures, that the OAE patent itself delayed the development of OAE technology. This is untrue. What delayed the commercial development of OAE technology throughout the 1980s was a combination of two things: skepticism and inertia within the audiological community and audiological ignorance, commercial protectionism, and underfunding within the commercial sector.

On the positive side, one British company did take the risk and developed the world's first TEOAE system based on our laboratory system. This was the Peters Ltd. UK's AP200 instrument described in Figure 1–21B and launched in 1985! Unfortunately, they sold only 7 units before going bank-rupt—perhaps justifying the timidness of U.S. manufacturers!

Although the 1980s was a static time for commercial instrument devel-opment, a large amount of OAE research involving many laboratories took place, much of it involving DPOAEs. There was comparatively less clinical research. In my own laboratory, important laboratory work was performed by Ann Brown exploring the properties of DPOAEs (e.g., Kemp & Brown, 1984; Brown & Kemp, 1984, 1985) and a wide range of techniques were evolved—not all yet in clinical use. DPOAEs began to be explored for clin-ical purposes (Kemp, Bray, Alexander, & Brown, 1986; Lonsbury-Martin & Martin, 1989). TEOAEs, on the other hand, began to be used for screening, beginning with the work of Johnsen in 1983 and including the work of Stevens et al. (1987), Bonfils, Uziel, and Pujol (1988), and Lutman (1989), all four with different locally made OAE systems.

The absence of a commercial OAE instrument limited research to those able to design and construct their own. Results were difficult to com-pare because system characteristics differed so widely. This was unsatis-factory. By 1988, and with no sign of commercial interest in sight, the Insti-tute of Laryngology and Otology (ILO) sanctioned the formation of Oto-dynamics Ltd. to develop and manufacture TE and DPOAE systems based on its own laboratory designs. The philosophy of this move was to "pub-lish" our research work as hardware in order to promote wider interest in the clinical use of OAEs.

Peter Bray of the ILO transferred the ILO laboratory TEOAE system functions—a set of amplifiers and a digital averager onto a PC card—with software to create the first commercially available OAE screening product—the ILO88 (Bray & Kemp, 1987; Bray, 1989). The ILO88 system (see Figure 1–21C) was designed to be a screening instrument but with full data analy-sis and research level documentation. As such it was adopted for the now famous Rhode Island Hearing Assessment project (White & Behrens, 1993). The success of TEOAEs in the Rhode Island program helped to promote universal newborn screening in the United States and elsewhere in the world (NIH, 1993; Davis, et al., 1997). Today there are probably 3,000–4,000 systems around the world, some up to 10 years old, collecting compatible TEOAE data. The ILO system was further developed to record and analyze both TE and DPOAEs (see Figure 1–20 and Kemp, 1997b).

During the 1990s, other laboratories followed the lead of the ILO and looked for opportunities to transfer their experience with OAEs into com-mercial products. The Virtual 330 DPOAE instrument, launched in 1990, was based on the laboratory research of Brenda and Glen Martin at Baylor College. The Cubdis DPOAE system was based on OAE work by Jont Allen at Bell Labs. More recently, Biologic has introduced an OAEs system (Scout) based on work by Steve Neely at the Boy's Town Institute and having DP and TEOAE potential. Instruments of nonacademic origin have also appeared, the first being created in Europe by Madsen—the Celeste DP and TEOAE system launched in 1993 and then the Welch Allyn GSI60 DP-only system, launched in 1995.

A central feature of any OAE instrument is its ability to discriminate between stimulus, noise, and OAE. Recognizing OAEs is straightforward, since they have a number of physical characteristics not shared by noise, stimuli, or other artifacts. As we have seen, true TE and DPOAEs have 2–12 ms latency, 99% reproducibility, strong nonlinearity, and exhibit sharply tuned suppressability. Comprehensive OAE examination would test for all of these factors to ensure the validity of any OAE. The ILO88/92 series of instruments test for reproducibility, latency, and nonlinearity in both TEOAE and DPOAE responses. Many other machines do not. Three tones are of course necessary to test the tuned suppressability of an OAE and this is so far only available on research machines such as the ILO96. The concern with clinical DPOAE measurements is that there may be some level of stimulation where passive distortion not related to the transduction process is created by the ear. This has been seen in small rodents but rarely in humans. Nevertheless, increasing stimulation for a moderately to severely impaired patient's ear will eventually give rise to a distortion signal, if not from the ear then from the probe. Rather than set an arbitrary upper limit for DPOAE stimulation (some adopt a cautious limit of 70 dB SPL), it would seem much better to test for the cochlear origin of any doubtful DPOAE by checking latency and, ideally, tuning.

OAE technology development is already dividing in two. The rapid growth of universal newborn hearing screening has created a need for smaller, portable and automatic scoring OAE systems. Figure 1–21D illustrates our laboratory's device—the EchoCheck—which uses nonlinear and reproducibility validation. Other hand-held devices include the Biologic "Audx" DP system and the Fischer Zoth "EchoScreen" TEOAE unit. Part of the success of these devices is their speed and convenience compared to ABR.

Newborn OAEs are virtually detectable in real time. The CD included with this book contains a program called REALTIME which will collect TEOAEs in combination with any ILO OAE system (ILO88, 88DP, Echoport, etc.) (Bray, 1998). By relaxing the normally conservative validation procedure this program shows TEOAEs "live" on the screen. This contrasts with ABR signal recording in which averaging is always necessary for recovery because the ABR signal is only a small part (1/50th) of the continuous EEG activity.

As screening devices become smaller, faster, easier to use, more reliable, and cheaper, it remains to be seen which technology will emerge as most effective in this form. It is also unclear right now what frequency range and frequency resolution will finally be accepted as adequate for newborn screening.

Clinical devices have yet to mature. Today's clinical commercial OAE instruments perform basically the same measurement made in research laboratories 15 and 20 years ago, albeit more conveniently. With these facilities, OAEs provide an indispensable objective test of cochlear status although we have yet to discover how to use them to really quantify the state of health of the cochlea. There is more to learn about OAEs.

## OAEs IN THE FUTURE

How could the clinical use of OAEs expand in the future and will it happen? In so far as the cochlea is the site of most sensory hearing problems and OAEs tell us directly about conditions inside the cochlea, we should expect to be able to learn much more from OAEs. Early hopes that OAEs would replace the audiogram were ill-founded. The clinical use at present is limited to essentially a half-octave by half-octave, normal/abnormal test of cochlear function. But current research on OAEs promises much more.

To take just one example, we can use OAEs to study the dynamics of cochlea maintenance. The maintenance of optimum conditions to give maximum sensitivity in the healthy ear clearly involves a number of systems, including the cochlear efferent system (e.g., Collet et al., 1992). When the cochlea is disturbed, corrective activity is initiated to restore equilibrium. The time course of the recovery from induced changes in OAE production reveals the status of the whole control system. The use of OAEs to show the depression in the travelling wave that accompanies noise induced threshold shift is long established. Exponential OAE recovery is seen with temporary threshold shift (Kemp, 1982). But in Figure 1–22A, we see the subtle effect of very mild acoustic stress in an oscillatory recovery of a cochlea to a mild noise exposure traced out by an SOAE. Exactly the same recovery dynamics are seen in the recovery of threshold (Figure 1–22B). What if this control system was impaired, but not the cochlea? Would it induce or allow cochlear pathology to develop? Suppose the control system was active and powerful. Would it hide the onset of cochlear pathology, keeping threshold apparently normal until its control was exhausted? Could OAEs dynamics measured clinically be used to predict future hearing losses and noise susceptibility? These are questions worth considering. Answers will require much more advanced OAE systems than are available today.

If we can ensure that auditory research labs and the audiological instrument manufacturing industry are better linked than in the past, we could see rapid evolution of audiometric instrumentation of all kinds. The

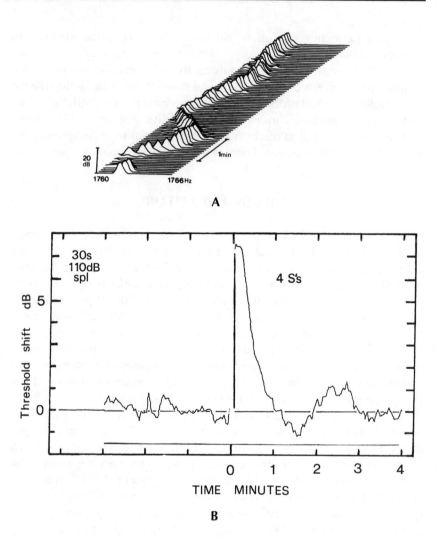

**Figure 1–22.** A time series of spectra of a spontaneous OAE revealing the undulations in cochlear mechanics following a brief and mild acoustic insult. Starting at the near trace, the normal spontaneous emission is seen as a peak at 1762 Hz. The break indicates the abolition of the SOAE during a 45-second exposure to a 100-Hz tone at 110 dB SPL. After the end of the exposure, the SOAE returns at a lower frequency. Its frequency rises and its strength grows. Both exceed the original values approximately 90 seconds after the end of the exposure. The SOAE returns to normal by executing an oscillatory recovery path. The same oscillatory recovery is seen in noise induced threshold shifts (from Kemp, 1986). **B.** Below shows averaged automatic threshold between 1 and 1.7 kHz in 4 subjects before and after a 30-second exposure to tones below 1 kHz. Hyperacusis occurs 90 seconds after the termination of the exposure—exactly when SOAE production peaked. The same oscillatory recovery is seen.

next few years could see vast improvements in the quantification OAEs with a switch from ear canal sound pressure to energy absorption as the primary measure. Tympanic reflectance measurement will reduce variance introduced by the ear canal, middle ear, and other acoustic factors (Keefe, 1991). Stimuli for OAE measurement will become much more complex (e.g., see Thornton, 1993) and dynamic, moving away from the click or tone pair choice of today. Computer-controlled complex stimuli will explore and adapt to individual ear characteristics, tracing suppression and tuning to produce an "acoustic scan" of the cochlea. Multiple parameters will be integrated to "type" cochlear status rather than bombard us with engineering graphs. Instruments will no longer measure just one DP, but all DPs and stimulus frequency emissions, too, not only to tones and clicks, but also to complex sounds. OAE latency measurement and suppression tuning curves tracing will be an integral part of the recording. Factors such as "hair cell nonlinearity profiles," "noise recovery time constants," and "efferent susceptibility" will be measured and discussed as part of in-depth auditory health checks for all.

To ensure these developments do happen, we need to learn a lesson from the last 50 years of hearing research. The rate of progress in audiology is limited only by the degree of imagination and open-mindedness the audiological community applies to new ideas and by the degree of determination and energy that we apply to exploring and understanding the ear.

**Acknowledgements:** The author gratefully acknowledges the contribution of his scientific collaborators at the Institute of Laryngology and Otology (ILO) including (in order of participation since 1975) Tony Martin, Patricia Lewis, Stewart Anderson, Lilly Alexander, Ann Brown, Peter Bray, Siobhan Ryan, David Brass, Mark Souter, Annie Moulin, Cliodna O Mahoney, and Bo Engdahl. Within the Institute, the engineering of experimental equipment and the development of the early OAE instruments owe everything to Peter Bray, David Brass, Rudolph Chum, and Jim Cousins.

During the course of work on OAEs we have received funding from the Royal National Throat Nose and Ear Hospital, the Hearing Research Trust, the Medical Research Council, and the Welcome Trust.

On behalf of the Institute of Laryngology and Otology and of the Royal National Throat Nose and Ear Hospital, the author thanks the manufacturers of commercial DP and TEOAEs instruments, who have respected the OAE patent and supported hearing research by paying royalties on OAE equipment sales. The contributing companies are Otodynamics Ltd., Madsen Danavox, Etymotics Inc, Fischer Zoth GmbH, and Hortmann GmbH. The author also thanks the other manufactures of OAE instruments in the U.S.A. for informing him of their expert opinion that the clinical uses and technology of DPOAEs were well known before the discovery of OAEs. He cordially invites them to read this chapter and reconsider!

# REFERENCES

Allen, J. B., & Fahey, P. F. (1992). Using acoustic distortion products to measure the cochlear amplifier gain on the basilar membrane. *Journal of the Acoustical Society of America, 92*, 178-188.

Békèsy, G. von. (1960). *Experiments in hearing.* New York: McGraw-Hill.

Bialek, W., & Wit, H. P. (1984). Quantum limits to oscillator stability: Theory and experiments on acoustic emissions from the human ear. *Phys Lett, 104A*, 173-178.

Bonfils, P., Uziel, A., & Pujol, R. (1988). Screening for auditory dysfunction in infants by evoked otoacoustic emissions. *Archives of Otolaryngology—Head and Neck Surgery, 114*, 887-890.

Brass, D., & Kemp, D. T. (1993). Analyses of Mossbauer mechanical measurements indicate that the cochlea is mechanically active. *Journal of the Acoustical Society of America, 93*, 1502-1515.

Brass, D., & Kemp, D.T. (1998). Visualising the cochlear traveling wave. Computer program (CD) In: *Otoacoustic emissions.* San Diego: Singular Publishing Group.

Bray, P. (1989). *Click evoked otoacoustic emissions and the development of a clinical otoacoustic hearing test instrument.* London University, PhD Thesis.

Bray, P. (1998). *REALTIME—realtime OAE display software for ILO systems.* [Software]. CD, San Diego: Singular Publishing Group/Otodynamics ltd.

Bray, P., & Kemp, D. T. (1987). An advanced cochlear echo technique suitable for infant screening. *British Journal of Audiology, 21*, 191-204.

Brink, G., van den. (1970). *Frequency analysis and periodicity detection in hearing.* (Sythoff, Leiden) pp 362-374.

Brown, A. M., & Kemp, D. T. (1984). Suppressibility of the $2f_1$-$f_2$ stimulated acoustic emissions in gerbil and man. *Hearing Research, 13*, 29-37.

Brown, A. M., & Kemp, D. T. (1985). Intermodulation distortion in the cochlea: Could basal vibration be the major cause of round window CM distortion? *Hearing Research, 19*, 191-198.

Brown, A. M., & Williams, D. M. (1993). A second filter in the cochlea. In H. Duifhuis, J. W. Horst, P. van Dijk, & S. M. van Netten (Eds.), *Proceedings of the International Symposium Biophysics of Hair Cell Sensory Systems*, London.

Collet, L., Veuillet, E., Bene, J., & Morgon, A. (1992). Effects of contralateral white noise on click-evoked emissions in normal and sensorineural ears: Towards an exploration of the medial olivocochlear system. *Audiology, 31*, 1-7.

Dallos, P. J. (1966). On the generation of odd-fractional subharmonics. *Journal of the Acoustical Society of America, 40*, 1381-1391.

Dallos, P.J. (1973). *The auditory periphery: Biophysics and physiology* (pp. 448-464). New York: Academic Press.

Davis, A., Bamford, J., et al. (1997). A critical review of the role of neonatal hearing screening in the detection of congenital hearing impairment. In U.K. Deptartment of Health, *Health Technology Assessment, 1*, (10).

de Boer, E. (1980). Nonlinear interactions and the "Kemp echo." *Hearing Research, 2*, 519-526.

Flottorp, G. (1953). Pure tone tinnitus evoked by acoustic stimulation: The idiophone effect. *Acta Otolaryngologica, 43*, 396-415.

Glanville, J. D., Coles, R. R. R., & Sullivan, B. M. (1971). A family with high-tonal objective tinnitus. *Journal of Laryngology and Otology*, 85, 1-10.

Gold, T. (1948). Hearing II. The physical basis of the action of the cochlea. *Proceeding of the Royal Society of Biological Sciences, 135*, 492-498.

Gold, T. (1989) Historical background to the proposal 40 years ago, of an active model for cochlear frequency analysis. In J. P. Wilson & D. T. Kemp (Eds.), *Cochlear mechanisms: Structure, function and models.* (pp. 299-306). London: Plenum.

Gold, T., & Pumphrey, R. J. (1948). Hearing. I: The cochlea as a frequency analyzer. *Proceeding of the Royal Society of Biological Sciences, 135*, 462-491.

Goldstein, J. L. (1967). Auditory nonlinearity. *Journal of the Acoustical Society of America, 41*, 676-689.

Johnsen, N. J., Bagi, P., & Elberling, C. (1983). Evoked acoustic emissions from the human ear. III. Findings in neonates. *Scandinavian Audiology, 12*, 17-24.

Keefe, D. H. (1991). Effects of external and middle ear characteristics on otoacoustic emissions. *Abstracts of International Sympiosium on Otoacoustic Emissions*, Kansas City, Missouri.

Kemp, D. T. (1970). *Observation on the resonator-type oscillations of the electromagnetic field in the cavity between the earth and the ionosphere.* PhD thesis, London University.

Kemp, D. T. (1971). The global location of large lightning discharges from single station observations of ELF disturbances in the Earth-ionosphere cavity. *Journal of Atmospheric and Terrestrial Physics, 33*, 919-927.

Kemp, D. T., & Martin, J. A. M. (1976). *Active resonant systems in audition*, XIII International Congress of Audiology, Firenze October 1976 Abstracts page 64 (reproduced as an appendix to this chapter).

Kemp, D. T. (1978a). Hearing Faculty test device. U.K. provisional patent No. 5467/78.

Kemp, D. T. (1978b, April). *Acoustic resonances originating inside the cochlea.* Presentation at the meeting of the British Society of Audiology. Reproduced here in Appendix C of this chapter.

Kemp, D. T. (1978c). Stimulated acoustic emissions from within the human auditory system. *Journal of the Acoustical Society of America, 64*, 1386-1391.

Kemp, D. T. (1979a). Evidence of mechanical nonlinearity and frequency selective wave amplification in the cochlea. *Archives of Otorhinolaryngology, 224*, 37-45.

Kemp, D. T. (1979b). The evoked cochlear mechanical response and the auditory microstructure—Evidence for a new element in cochlear mechanics. *Scandinavian Audiology, 9*, 35-47.

Kemp, D. T. (1981). Physiologically active cochlear micromechanics One source of tinnitus. In: *Tinnitus.* Ciba Foundation Sympiosium, D Evered, G Lawrenson (Eds). (pp54- 81). London: Pitman Books Ltd.

Kemp, D. T. (1982). Cochlear echoes: Implications for noise-induced hearing loss. In R. P. Hamerick, D. Henderson, & R. Salvi (Eds.), *New perspectives on noise-induced hearing loss* (pp. 189-207). New York: Raven.

Kemp, D. T. (1986). Otoacoustic emissions, travelling waves and cochlear mechanisms. *Hearing Research, 22*, 95-104.

Kemp, D.T. (1997a). Otoacoustic emissions in perspective. In R. M. Robinette & T. Glattke (Eds.), *Otoacoustic emissions—Clinical applications.* New York: Thieme.

Kemp, D. T. (1997b). *Understanding and using otoacoustic emissions*. Hatfield, UK: Otodynamics Ltd.

Kemp, D. T., Bray, P., Alexander, L., & Brown, A. M. (1986). Acoustic emission cochleography - Practical aspects. In G. Cianfrone & F. Grandori (Eds.), *Cochlear Mechanics and Otoacoustic Emissions, Scandinavian Audiology, 15*, (Suppl. 25) 71-96.

Kemp, D. T., Brass, D. N., & Souter, M. (1990). Observations on simultaneous SFOAE and DPOAE generation and suppression. In P. Dallos, C. D. Geisler, J. W. Matthews, M. A. Ruggero, & C. R. Steele (Eds.), *Mechanics and biophysics of hearing* (pp. 202-209). New York: Springer-Verlag.

Kemp, D. T., & Brown, A. M. (1983). A comparison of mechanical nonlinearities in the cochleae of man and gerbil from ear canal measurements. In R. Klinke & R. Hartmann (Eds.), *Hearing—Physiological bases and psychophysics* (pp. 82-88). Berlin: Springer-Verlag.

Kemp, D. T., & Brown, A. M. (1984). Ear canal acoustic and round window correlates of $2f_1-f_2$ distortion generated in the cochlea. *Hearing Research, 13*, 39-46.

Kemp, D. T., & Brown, A. M. (1986). Wideband analysis of otoacoustic intermodulation. In J. B. Allen, J. L. Hall, A. Hubbard, S. T. Neeley, & A. Tubis (Eds.), *Peripheral auditory mechanisms* (pp. 306-313). New York: Springer-Verlag.

Kemp, D. T., & Sivanessan, S. (1998). Three tone interactions in the human ear. (in preparation)

Kim, D. O. (1980a). Chairman: Transcript of the mid symposium discussion. Nonlinear and active mechanical processes in the cochlear. *Hearing Research, 2*, 581-587.

Kim, D. O. (1980b). Cochlear mechanics: Implications of electrophysiological and acoustical observations. *Hearing Research, 2*, 297-317.

Kim, D. O., Seigel, J. H., & Molnar, C. E. (1977). Cochlear distortion products: Inconsistency with linear motion of the cochlear partition. *Journal of the Acoustical Society of America, 61*, S2(A).

Kimberley, P., Brown, D. K., & Allen J. B. (1997). Distortion product emissions and sensori neural hearing loss. In R. M. Robinette & T. Glattke (Eds.), *Otoacoustic emissions—Clinical applications* (pp. 306-313). New York: Thieme.

Lonsbury-Martin, B. L. & Martin, G. K. (1989). Clinical applications of distortion-product emissions. *Asha Abstracts, 31*, 142.

Lutman, M. E. (1989). Evoked otoacoustic emissions in adults: Implications for screening. *Audiology Practice, 6*, 6-8.

Moulin, A., & Kemp, D. T. (1996). Multicomponent acoustic distortion product otoacoustic emission phase in humans II. Implications for distortion product otoacoustic emission generation. *Journal of the Acoustical Society of America, 100*, 1640-1662.

NIH. (1993). *National Institutes of Health Consensus Statement on early detection of hearing impairment in infants and young children* (pp. ii, 1-24). Washington, DC: Author.

Norton, S. J., & Neely, S. T. (1987). Tone-burst-evoked otoacoustic emissions from normal-hearing subjects. *Journal of the Acoustical Society of America, 81*, 1860-1872.

O Mahoney, C., & Kemp, D. T. (1995). Distortion product otoacoustic emission daly measurement in human ears. *Journal of the Acoustical Society of America, 97*, 3721-3735.

Rhode, W. S. (1971). Observations of the vibration of the basilar membrane in squirrel monkey using the Mossbauer technique. *Journal of the Acoustical Society of America, 49,* 1218-1321.

Stevens, J. C., Webb, H. D., Smith, M. F., Buffin, J. T., & Ruddy, H. (1987). A comparison of oto-acoustic emissions and brain stem electric response audiometry in the normal newborn and babies admitted to a special care baby unit. *Clinical Physics and Physiological Measurement, 8,* 95-104.

Thomas, L. B. (1975). Microstructure of the pure tone threshold. *Journal of the Acoustical Society of America, 57,* 26-27.

Thornton, A. R. D. (1993). High rate otoacoustic emissions. *Journal of the Acoustical Society of America, 94,* 132-136.

Tubis, A., & Talmadge, G. L. (1998). Ear canal reflectance in the presence of spontaneous otoacoustic emissions. *Journal of the Acoustical Society of America, 103,* 454-465.

Ward, W. D. (1955). Tonal monaural diplacusis. *Journal of the Acoustical Society of America, 27,* 365-372.

Wegel, R. L. (1931). A study of tinnitus. *Archives of Otolaryngology, 14,* 158-165.

Welch, Allyn. (1995). A complete guide to otoacoustic emissions. Welch Allyn, NH: Author.

White, K. R., & Behrens, T. R. (1993). The Rhode Island Hearing Assessment Project: Implications for universal newborn screening. *Seminars in Hearing, 14,* (1).

Wilson, J. P. (1980). Evidence for a cochlear origin for acoustic re-emissions, threshold fine- structure and tonal tinnitus. *Hearing Research, 2,* 233-252.

Wit, H. P., & Ritsma, R. J. (1980). On the mechanism of the evoked cochlear mechanical response. In G. van den Brink, & F. A. Bilson (Eds.) *Psychophysical, physiological and behavioural studies in hearing* (pp. 53-63). Delft, the Netherlands: Delft University Press.

# APPENDIX A

## SOFTWARE ON CD

There are three programs on the CD, DIEP1D and REALTIME, and ILONS

DIEP1D was written by David Brass, as a teaching aid for the Master's courses in Audiology Science and Audiological Mediciine held at the Institute of Laryngolgoy and Otology. It is a spinoff from his own research work on the cochlea and OAEs and demonstrates the travelling wave in the cochlea.

REALTIME was written by Peter Bray, designer of the ILO88 OAE system. This program allows real time display of TEOAEs if any ILO system is fitted to the computer. The software is not intended for clinical use but rather as a research and teaching aid.

ILONS can be used to review TEOAE data files and simulate an OAE recording session.

## Use of the Cochlear Travelling Wave Program on CD

This program demonstrates the general form of traveling waves on the cochlea and is based on the work of Deipendal. The program was written by David Brass of the Institute of Laryngology and Otology. Although it presents a useful visual image of many aspects of the cochlear traveling wave, it is not intended to be a quantitative tool for research.

In this graphic presentation, the cochlea is represented as being straight. The horizontal line across the screen represents the basilar membrane, which is normally curled about three turns. The length is of the order of 3 cm. The leftmost part of the screen represents the base of the cochlea, the right the apex. The up-and-down motions in the form of waves on the basilar membrane would not in practice be visible in the real cochlea, because the true scale of motion is of subatomic dimensions for sounds near threshold. It never exceeds the dimensions of the cochlea cells for the most extreme levels of stimulation.

The program requires a minimum 486 processor. It can be launched from Windows (if a DIEP1D ICON appears on your screen), but actually runs under DOS by running the program DIEP1D. See the CD label for installation details. On starting the program, a text instruction screen is shown. You can run the model right away or take the option to change stimulus and damping parameters. You may also inspect all the parameters used with the model. Many of these parameters should not be changed as they may result in unpredictable results. The parameters of most interest are the frequencies and amplitudes of the two tones notionally presented to the model cochlea. Using the default settings, press the ESCAPE key and observe the motion of the basilar membrane gradually increase and differentiate into two peaks. Use the SPACE key to pause the travelling wave. The default settings are for two tones at 4 kHz and 6 kHz of equal input intensity. The program will run at different speeds, depending on the speed of the computer processor. The real time represented on the display is shown on the top left. Waves will move from left to right in sinusoidal fashion, growing in intensity toward the peak for each frequency. The travelling waves freeze when the termination time is reached. A number of revealing experiments can be performed using this program.

To demonstrate the frequency resolution of the cochlea, tones at different frequencies can be applied. When these frequencies become closer, a point will be reached where the component frequencies cannot be resolved as two separate peaks of the travelling wave. Only one coalesced peak is seen. Obviously, the sharpness of the individual peaks determines this limiting resolution.

The resolution of the model cochlea is determined by the mechanical properties of its components and the degree of damping, or energy loss associated with the model structure. The damping for the model can be changed by pressing "D" and using the cursor keys. The default value is 0.40. Increasing the damping parameter will reduce the size and sharpness of the travelling wave peaks. In this case, the resolution of the cochlea will be reduced, and its sensitivity, represented by the input amplitude needed to achieve a given level of excitation within the cochlea, will also be reduced. Decreasing the damping factor will result in sharper and much larger travelling wave peaks for a given stimulus input. The resolution of the cochlea will also be greatly enhanced. However, if the damping is made too low the cochlea model becomes unstable. This may crash the computer program.

Each time the DIEP1D program is terminated in the normal way (QUIT), a configuration file is written (ending with .DEF), which contains the last settings of the various parameters. The default settings can be restored by pressing R at the second screen. Unfortunately, it is not possible to answer questions about this program or its operation. It was written purely for demonstration teaching purposes at the Institute of Laryngology and Otology. The source code is not available. (Copyright D. Brass, 1995, 8.)

## Use of REALTIME TEOAE software

This program will show TEOAEs live on the screen.

It is necessary to have an ILO OAE system installed on your PC. See the CD label for installation instructions. RUN REALTIME or click on the REALTIME icon if it appears on your screen. On first calling, select the ILO system you have installed. Fit the probe to an ear with strong OAEs and watch the emissions. Save waveforms to lower trace with the S key. Check reproducibility by overlaying traces. Adjust the artifact reject level with the cursor keys. (Written by P. Bray, Copyright 1994 Otodynamics Ltd.)

## Use of ILOVS

Run this program from the CD. Select TEOAE, then "files," then "review." Select one of the many data files for review. After selection, go to "tests" to simulate a recording session.

## APPENDIX B*

*Presented at the XIII International Congress of Audiology, Firenze, Italy October 1976
Abstracts, page 64

## Active Resonant Systems in Audition

### D.T. Kemp and J.A. Martin

*The Royal National Throat, Nose & Ear Hospital, Nuffield Hearing and Speech Centre, Gray's Inn Road, London, WC1, England*

New psychophysical data will be presented relating to the microstructure of human audition at low stimulus levels. Very detailed measurements have been made of threshold, loudness, pitch, differential sensitivity, and critical ratio functions, with respect to frequency in several otologically normal subjects.

The occurrence of transient tonal tinnitus and associated distortions to pure tone reception have been correlated with a recurrent feature of the auditory microstructure.

The results obtained support the hypothesis that a framework of highly tuned ($Q > 50$) resonant systems assist in the reception of near-threshold sounds. The mechanism must be active and must be at least partly peripheral as it is susceptible to pressure changes in the cochlea.

# APPENDIX C

**\*Presented at the British Society of Audiology,** Short papers meeting, April 21st, 1978 [Abstracts].

## Acoustic Resonances Originating Inside the Cochlea\*

D.T. Kemp, Auditory Perception Research Laboratory, Royal National Throat, Nose and Ear Hospital, Gray's Inn Road, London, WC1X 8DA.

It is twenty years since Elliot (1958, *Nature, 181,* p. 1076) first reported "A Ripple Effect in the Audiogram," yet the existence of closely spaced and finely tuned sensitivity maxima in normal low level hearing has remained unexplained. Detailed psychophysical investigation has shown the phenomena to be too complex and too highly tuned to have their origin in passive acoustic, mechanical or hydromechanical resonances of the auditory system. An active mechanism that responds nonlinearly to stimulation, is indicated. The mechanism is sensitive to deflection of the ossicular chain (engineered by pneumatic pressure) and is also capable of continuous oscillation. An explanation involving standing waves in the cochlea, actively supported by the transduction process has been proposed (Kemp, 1976, British Society of Audiology, 6th October meeting, Guildford; 13th International Congress of Audiology, Florence).

A successful theoretical model has now been developed and will be briefly outlined. Physiological predictions, based on this model, have been tested and confirmed experimentally. This has led to the discovery of a mechanical cochlear response to be described for the first time (Kemp, 1978, *Journal of the Acoustical Society of America*, in press). New physiological techniques based on this response are providing a fresh avenue for the investigation of certain aspects of cochlear mechanics and the transduction mechanism at low stimulus levels. Preliminary results will be given. Clinical applications are anticipated (Kemp, 1978, National Research and Development Council, U.K. Patent Application 5467.78.)

# TRANSMITTERS IN THE COCHLEA
## The Quadratic Distortion Product and Its Time Varying Response May Reflect the Function of ATP in the Cochlea

*Richard P. Bobbin, Ph.D.*
*Chu Chen, Ph.D.*
*Anastas P. Nenov, M.D., Ph.D.*
*Ruth A. Skellett, Ph.D.*
Kresge Research Laboratory of the South
Department of Otorhinolaryngology and Biocommunication
Louisiana State University Medical Center
New Orleans, Louisiana

Evidence is accumulating to indicate that extracellular adenosine 5'-triphosphate (ATP) may function as a neurotransmitter, neuromodulator, mitogen, and cytotoxin (Burnstock, 1990; Collo, North, Kawashima, Merlo-Pich, Neidhart, Surprenant, & Buell, 1996; Wang, Huang, Heller, & Heppel, 1994; Zoeteweij, Van de Water, De Bont, & Nagelkerke, 1996). ATP receptors appear to belong to one superfamily that is distinct from other receptors. Currently both functional and molecular biology classifications of ATP receptors are being used. The receptors that act by way of a ligand-gated ion channel (ionotropic receptors) are classified as P2X and to date seven have been sequenced and cloned ($P2X_1$-$P2X_7$). Those receptors that act by way of a ligand-activated G protein (metabotropic) are classified as P2Y and currently five have been identified.

## THE FUNCTION OF ATP IN THE COCHLEA

Bobbin and Thompson (1978) first suggested that ATP and ATP receptors may have a function in the cochlea by demonstrating that extracellular application of ATP to the cells of the cochlea by perfusion of the perilymph compartment affected the function of the cochlea as monitored by a change in the compound action potential of the auditory nerve. Subsequently, ATP-induced alterations in activity of the afferent nerve innervating lateral line hair cells was demonstrated (Bobbin, Morgan, & Bledsoe, 1979; Mroz & Sewell, 1989). At the single cell level, ATP has been shown to induce ATP receptor activation (both metabotropic and ionotropic) in several cell types in the cochlea. ATP receptors have been functionally identified in outer hair cells ([OHCs]; Ashmore & Ohmori, 1990; Chen, Nenov, & Bobbin, 1995; Chen, Nenov, Norris, & Bobbin, 1995; Housley, Greenwood, & Ashmore, 1992; Ikeda, Saito, Nishiyama, & Takasaka, 1991; Kakehata, Nakagawa, Takasaka, & Akaike, 1993; Kujawa, Erostegui, Fallon, Crist, & Bobbin, 1994; Nakagawa, Akaike, Kimitsuki, Komune, & Arima, 1990; Shigemoto & Ohmori, 1990); inner hair cells (IHCs; Dulon, Mollard, & Aran, 1991; Suga-sawa, Erostegui, Blanchet, & Dulon, 1996); Deiters' cells (Dulon, 1995; Dulon, Moataz, & Mollard, 1993); Hensen's cells (Dulon, Moataz, & Mollard, 1993), and cells of the stria vascularis (Liu, Kozakura, & Marcus, 1995; Munoz, Thorne, Housley, & Billett, 1995; Munoz, Thorne, Housley, Billett, & Battersby, 1995; Suzuki et al., 1995; Wangemann, 1995; White et al., 1995).

At the present time, the functions of ATP receptors in the cochlea are unknown (Bobbin, 1996; Eybalin, 1993). Deiters' cells may respond to extracellular ATP with a change in stiffness and through this mechanism ATP may be involved in modulating cochlear mechanics (Bobbin, Chen, Skellett, & Fallon, 1997; Dulon, 1995; Skellett, Chen, Fallon, Nenov, & Bobbin, 1997). ATP receptors on the stria may regulate the endocochlear potential (Suzuki et al., 1995; Wangemann, 1995). The ionotropic receptors on OHCs may be involved in transduction, as they appear to be located on the scala media surface of the OHCs (Housley et al., 1992; Mockett, Housley, & Thorne, 1994; Mockett, Bo, Housley, Thorne, & Burnstock, 1995). ATP may act as a cytotoxin, killing cells when exposed to large amounts of ATP possibly released from killer lymphocytes or cells in the organ of Corti during noise exposure (Bobbin, Chu, Skellett, Campbell, & Fallon, 1997; Chu et al., 1997). ATP may also act as a mitogen, stimulating the proliferation of fibrocytes in the spiral ligament (Bobbin et al., 1997; Chu et al., 1997).

## THE FUNCTION OF ATP IN THE ORGAN
## OF CORTI: A HYPOTHESIS

One working hypothesis in our laboratory is that endogenous *ATP modulates cochlear mechanics in the organ of Corti through an action on ionotropic receptors on Deiters' cells.* To prove that any endogenous substance has such a role, a set of criteria has to be met (as discussed in Bobbin, Bledsoe, Winbery, & Jenison, 1985). Among these criteria are: (1) the exogenous application of the substance should *mimic* the effects of the endogenously released substance; (2) drugs that block the effects of the endogenous substance should also *block* the effects when the substance is applied exogenously; (3) the substance should be *released* into the extracellular space on stimulation of the cells of origin; (4) the substance should be *synthesized* in the cells from which it is released; (5) a mechanism for *terminating* the action of the substance should exist; and (6) the *receptor protein and mRNA* for the protein must be present in the cells where the substance is thought to act.

# EVIDENCE FOR THE HYPOTHESIS

To monitor cochlear mechanics, we use distortion product otoacoustic emissions (DPOAEs), as they are generated in part by, and appear to be a reflection of, the active cochlear mechanics in the organ of Corti. Active mechanics involve the OHC-Deiters' cell complex. OHCs shorten and lengthen in response to changes in their resting membrane potential (Bobbin, 1996; Brownell, 1996). Because the OHCs are held by the Deiters' cells at their base and at their apex, the Deiters' cells can alter or modify the movement of the OHCs by a change in their own stiffness. Dulon, Blanchet, and Laffon (1994) demonstrated a change in the stiffness of Deiters' cells in response to a change in intracellular $Ca^{2+}$. We assume that any change in the mechanics of this cellular complex will be reflected in changes in the DPOAEs (as discussed by Frank & Kossl, 1996). Thus, when we refer to changes in cochlear mechanics, we will mean a change in mechanics as monitored through changes in DPOAEs.

## Action of Exogenously Applied ATP: The Mimic Criteria

To test the hypothesis, our first goal was to determine if we could detect an action of exogenously applied ATP on cochlear mechanics as monitored by DPOAEs (Bobbin, Fallon, Crist, Kujawa, & Erostegui, 1993; Kujawa, Fallon, & Bobbin, 1993; Kujawa, Erostegui, Fallon, Crist, & Bobbin, 1994). To accomplish this we perfused the perilymph scalae of guinea pigs with artificial perilymph containing ATP and monitored the cubic DPOAE ($2f_1-f_2$) in the ear canal. We placed the drug in the perilymph as it has long been known that drugs readily diffuse from the perilymph through the basilar membrane to distribute in the fluid surrounding OHCs and Deiters' cells. As shown in Figure 2–1, ATP induced a small suppression of the cubic DPOAEs. It was possible the response to ATP was slight because ATP is

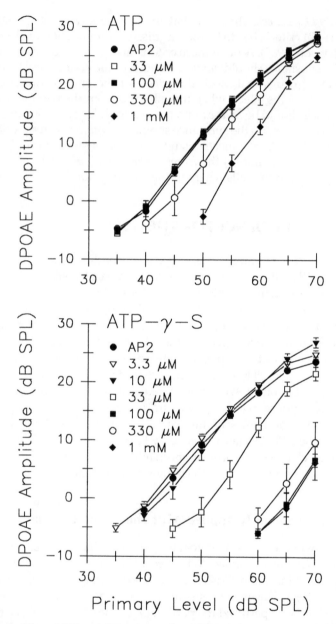

**Figure 2–1.** Effect of ATP and ATP-γ-S on cubic ($2f_1-f_2$) DPOAE responses recorded from the external ear canal as a function of stimulus intensity. Shown in each panel are amplitude growth functions recorded after predrug artificial perilymph perfusions (AP2) and after perfusion with increasing concentrations of ATP and ATP-γ-S. Data are represented as means ± SE across five animals. (From "Effects of Adenosine 5'-triphosphate and Related Agonists on Cochlear Function," by S. G. Kujawa, C. Erostegui, M. Fallon, J. Crist, and R. P. Bobbin, 1994. *Hearing Research, 76,* pp. 87–100. Reprinted with permission.)

rapidly metabolized by ectonucleotidases on the surface of the cells lining the perilymph compartment such as OHCs (Vlajkovic, Thorne, Munoz, & Housley, 1996). Therefore, we tested a chemical derivative of ATP, ATP-γ-S, that is resistant to the enzyme and therefore metabolized at a much slower rate than ATP. As shown in Figure 2–1, the ATP-γ-S was much more potent than ATP and almost abolished the cubic DPOAE at a concentration of 1 mM. Because the drug had little or no effect on the endocochlear potential (EP), it is reasonable to speculate that the drug acted on cells in the organ of Corti, particularly, the OHC-Deiters' cell complex.

Both OHCs and Deiters' cells have ATP receptors in their membranes. However, there is strong evidence that the ionotropic ATP receptors on OHCs are located on the endolymph side of the cells (Housley, Greenwood, & Ashmore, 1992; Mockett et al., 1994, 1995). Dulon (1995) and Dulon, Moataz, and Mollard (1993) suggested that the ATP receptors on Deiters' cells are located near the region where the cell contacts the base of the OHC, or on the perilymph side of the reticular lamina. If this is the case, then drugs such as ATP-γ-S, when placed in perilymph, therefore bathing the base and lateral walls but not the cuticular plate region of the OHCs, can only affect ionotropic ATP receptors on Deiters' cells, but not those on OHCs. These results on DPOAEs were the first evidence that our hypothesis may be correct (Criterion #1).

## Detection of an Action of Endogenously Released ATP on Mechanics: the Blockade Criterion

The results with agonists applied into the cochlea present evidence as to the effects of activation of the receptors but do not demonstrate that endogenous ATP is capable of having a similar role in normal or pathological physiology. To accomplish this task physiologists and pharmacologists have traditionally relied on the effects of antagonists. If an antagonist abolishes a physiological response, then this is taken as evidence that the blocked response was mediated by the endogenous substance (Criterion #2).

## Effect of Cibacron and Suramin on Cubic DPOAEs

Figure 2–2, taken from Kujawa, Fallon, and Bobbin (1994), shows that the ATP antagonist, cibacron blue (cibacron), when perfused through the perilymph compartment of guinea pig cochlea in a manner similar to the ATP perfusion, almost totally abolished the cubic DPOAE. This is evidence that cibacron blocked the actions of endogenous ATP at receptors on cells in the cochlea, that in turn prevented the production of normal DPOAEs. Parenthetically, it is not unusual for both an agonist such as ATP and an antagonist such as cibacron to exhibit similar effects when one is monitoring a remote response like the DPOAEs. For example, both ACh (an ago-

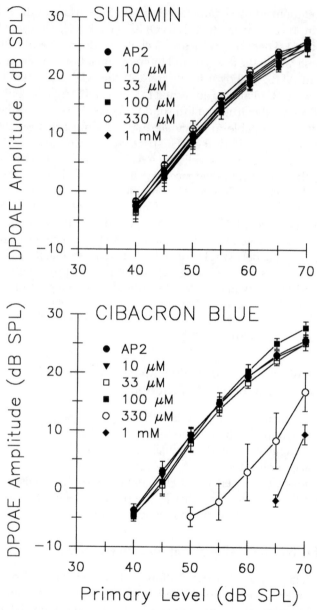

**Figure 2–2.** Effect of suramin and cibacron on the cubic $(2f_1-f_2)$ DPOAE as a function of stimulus intensity. Shown are amplitude growth functions recorded after predrug artificial perilymph perfusions (AP2) and after perfusion with increasing concentrations of suramin and cibacron. Data are represented as means Å SE across five animals for each drug. (From "ATP Antagonists Cibacron Blue, Basilen Blue and Suramin Alter Sound-Evoked Responses of the Cochlea and Auditory Nerve," by S. G. Kujawa, M. Fallon, and R. P. Bobbin, 1994. *Hearing Research, 78*, pp. 181–188. Reprinted with permission.)

nist) and curare (an antagonist) block the response of the efferents (Bobbin & Konishi, 1971a, 1971b, 1974). The results with cibacron blocking the generation of the cubic DPOAEs allow us to draw the tentative conclusion that endogenous release of ATP onto ATP receptors, possibly at the OHC-Deiters' cell complex, is necessary for the generation of the DPOAEs.

In the Kujawa, Fallon, and Bobbin (1994) study, suramin, an additional ATP antagonist, had no effect on the cubic DPOAE, even though it did abolish the compound action potential of the auditory nerve. This effect of suramin on the action potential may have been due to an action on glutamate, the afferent transmitter released from the inner hair cells (Aubert, Norris, & Guth, 1995; Bledsoe, Bobbin, & Puel, 1988; Bobbin et al., 1985). So the question remained as to whether suramin was indeed an ATP antagonist at the ATP receptors on OHCs and Deiters' cells.

## Action of ATP Antagonists (Cibacron, Suramin, and PPADS) at the Single Cell Level

To examine whether cibacron or suramin blocks the actions of ATP on OHCs and Deiters' cells, these cells were isolated from guinea pig cochlea and whole cell voltage clamp studies of the drugs were carried out. Under these conditions, the cells were studied directly and drug-induced changes in other properties of the cells were monitored.

As shown in Figure 2–3A, application of ATP to a Deiters' cell induced an inward current due to the ATP-induced activation of an ionotropic ATP receptor (Chen, LeBlanc, & Bobbin, 1997; Dulon, 1995). When suramin was applied together with ATP, the response to ATP was reduced (Figure 2–3A). This indicates that suramin is an antagonist of ATP at ATP receptors on these cells. Figure 2–3B and 2–3C illustrate the lack of effect of suramin on the currents induced by stepping the voltage of the cell to different values. Suramin induced no change in these voltage-induced currents indicating that suramin is specific for the ATP receptor protein and has no effect on the voltage activated ion channel proteins.

Results with cibacron were different from suramin. As shown in Figure 2–4A, cibacron was found to be a powerful blocker of ATP-induced currents, possibly more powerful than suramin. However, as shown in Figure 2–4B and 2–4C, cibacron also attenuated the voltage-induced outward potassium currents. Therefore, the effects of cibacron in vivo may be due to effects on both voltage-induced potassium currents and ATP-induced currents.

An additional ATP antagonist, pyridoxal-phosphate-6-azophenyl-2', 4'-disulphonic acid (PPADS), was examined at the single cell level and found to block ATP-induced currents (Figure 2–5). The block was slow to develop, as indicated by the much larger block of ATP after washing out the PPADS. To date, this block of ATP has not accompanied by other effects

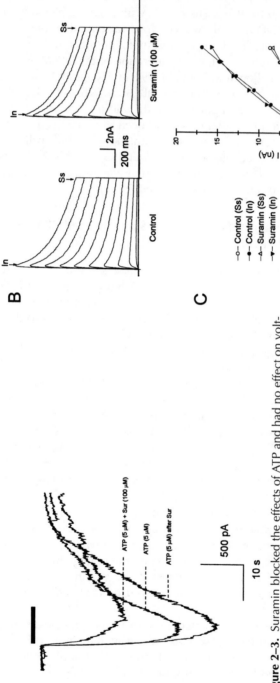

**Figure 2–3.** Suramin blocked the effects of ATP and had no effect on voltage induced currents in a Deiters' cell. **A.** ATP (5 μM)-induced currents are suppressed by suramin (100 μM). After washing out the suramin, the ATP response was greater than control. The cell was voltage clamped at −80 mV. **B.** Current voltage (I–V) relationships recorded from a Deiters' cell in the absence and presence of 100 μM suramin. The voltage command was stepped from −100 mV to +60 mV. **C.** I–V plots were constructed from the steady state (Ss) and instantaneous (In) values in B.

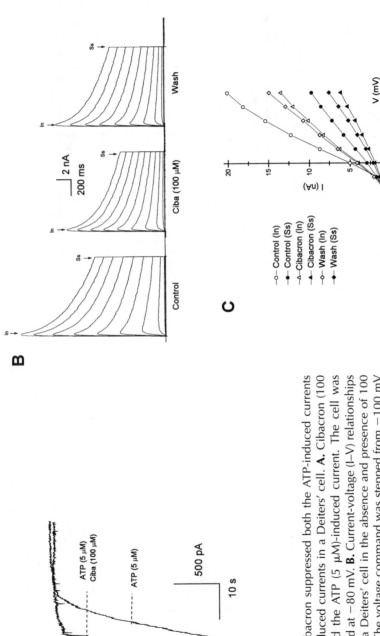

**Figure 2–4.** Cibacron suppressed both the ATP-induced currents and voltage-induced currents in a Deiters' cell. **A.** Cibacron (100 μM) suppressed the ATP (5 μM)-induced current. The cell was voltage clamped at −80 mV. **B.** Current-voltage (I–V) relationships recorded from a Deiters' cell in the absence and presence of 100 μM cibacron. The voltage command was stepped from −100 mV to +60 mV. **C.** I–V plots were constructed from the steady state (Ss) and instantaneous (In) values in B.

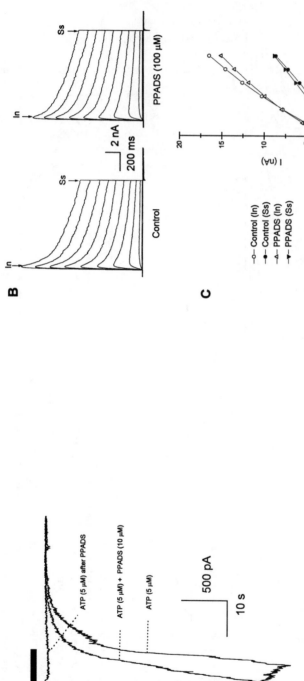

**Figure 2–5.** PPADS suppressed ATP-evoked currents with no effect on voltage-induced currents in a Deiters' cell. **A.** PPADS (10 μM) suppressed the ATP (5 μM)-evoked currents with a delay. The delay is observed as a greater blockade after washing out the PPADS than the amount of blockade when the PPADS was simultaneously applied with the ATP. The cell was voltage clamped at −80 mV. **B.** Current voltage (I–V) relationships recorded from a Deiters' cell in the absence and presence of 10 μM PPADS. The voltage command was stepped from −100 mV to +60 mV. **C.** I–V plots were constructed from the steady state (Ss) and instantaneous (In) values in B.

of PPADS, such as effects on voltage-induced potassium currents (Figure 2–5B and 2–5C). It appears that PPADS is a more potent ATP antagonist than either suramin or cibacron.

In summary, the only effect detected for both suramin and PPADS at the single cell level was a block of ATP-induced inward current. Cibacron, on the other hand, also affected voltage-induced potassium currents. Thus, the suppression of the cubic DPOAEs by cibacron, but not by suramin, possibly reflects the actions of cibacron on outward potassium currents.

## The Time Varying Amplitude Change in the Quadratic DPOAE ($f_2$–$f_1$)

After a period of silence, the quadratic DPOAE undergoes complex time varying changes in amplitude when monitored over minutes during continuous sound stimulation with moderate level primaries (Brown, 1988; Kirk & Johnstone, 1993; Kujawa, Fallon, & Bobbin, 1995; Kujawa, Fallon, Skellett, & Bobbin, 1996; Lowe and Robertson, 1995). The typical shape of response recorded from guinea pig cochlea is shown in Figure 2–6. Initially, it was thought that the efferent nerves innervating the cochlea were responsible for these changes in amplitude. However, Lowe and Robertson (1995) demonstrated conclusively that the efferents do not contribute to the amplitude change. Similar conclusions were reached by Kujawa et al. (1995) and Kujawa et al. (1996) who demonstrated that the amplitude change recorded from the guinea pig was not affected to a large extent by: TTX, a sodium channel antagonist; curare in concentrations that blocked the action of acetylcholine released by the efferents onto the OHCs; bicuculline, a GABA antagonist; and efferent sectioning. Thus it appears that neither the efferents nor any other kind of nerve action underlies the amplitude change. On the other hand, the amplitude was dramatically affected by drugs active at calcium channels such as nimodipine and Bay K (Kujawa et al., 1996).

## Effect of ATP Antagonists on the Time-Varying Amplitude Change of the Quadratic DPOAE

Others suggested that the quadratic DPOAE is a more sensitive indicator of the set point of the cochlear amplifier (Frank & Kossl, 1996). Thus the quadratic DPOAE may be a more sensitive indicator of the role of the OHC-Deiters' cell complex in the function of the cochlear mechanics. Therefore, we extended our pharmacological studies of the quadratic amplitude change to include the effects of ATP antagonists.

Figure 2–7 shows the effect of perfusing increasing concentrations of suramin through the perilymph compartment of guinea pig cochlea on the amplitude change in the quadratic DPOAE. Suramin blocked the decline in the amplitude of the quadratic DPOAE in a reversible manner without an

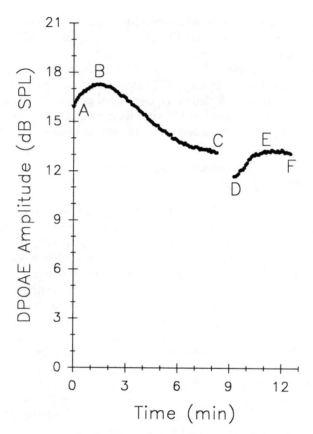

**Figure 2–6.** A typical example of the effect of continuous primary stimulation on cubic ($f_2$–$f_1$) DPOAE amplitude recorded from the ear canal immediately following a 15-min perfusion of the perilymph compartment with a second artificial perilymph (AP2) during which time the primaries were turned off and the animal kept in a sound attenuated environment. Each data point represents a 10-spectra average and required 5 s to complete. The break in the response amplitude trace (C–D) represents 1 min with no primary stimulation. Points A–F thus identified in each trace were used to calculate amplitude changes.

One hundred consecutive 10-spectra averages of distortion product amplitude were obtained during continuous primary stimulation ($f_1$ = 6.25 kHz, $f_2$ = 7.5 kHz, L1 = L2 = 60 dB SPL). Each of these averages required approximately 5 s to complete for a total of 500 s (8.3 min) of stimulation. The primary tones were then simultaneously turned off and there was a 1 min rest from primary stimulation. Following this rest, the primaries were reintroduced and 40 consecutive 10-spectra averages of distortion product amplitude were obtained (total time approximately 200 s or 3.3 min of stimulation).

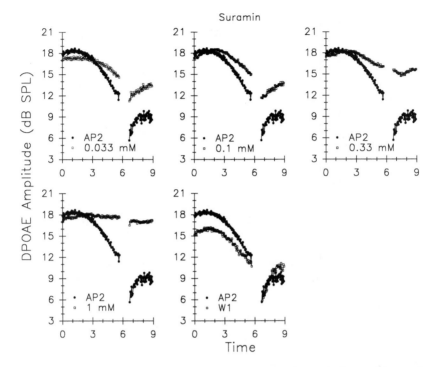

**Figure 2–7.** Suramin attenuates the decrease in the quadratic ($f_2 - f_1$) DPOAE amplitude induced by continuous primary stimulation. Shown are functions recorded in a typical animal after 15-min perfusions of pre-drug artificial perilymph perfusions (AP2), with increasing concentrations of suramin (0.033–1 mM), and a wash.

One hundred consecutive 5-spectra averages of distortion product amplitude were obtained during continuous primary stimulation ($f_1$ = 6.25 kHz, $f_2$ = 7.5 kHz, L1 = L2 = 60 dB SPL). Each of these averages required approximately 3.5 s to complete for a total of 350 s (5.83 min) of stimulation. The primary tones were then simultaneously turned off and there was a 1-min rest from primary stimulation. Following this rest, the primaries were reintroduced and 40 consecutive 5-spectra averages of distortion product amplitude were obtained (total time approximately 140 s or 2.3 min of stimulation).

effect on the initial starting value. Monitoring the amplitude of the quadratic DPOAE at various primary intensities indicated that the suramin shifted the function to the left (Figure 2–8). In contrast, the amplitude growth function of the cubic DPOAE was not altered (Figure 2–8).

When PPADS was tested in the same fashion as suramin, PPADS altered the amplitude change in a much more complex fashion than suramin (Figure 2–9). Low concentrations of PPADS (<0.10 mM) suppressed the initial value of the quadratic DPOAE at 60-dB primaries imme-

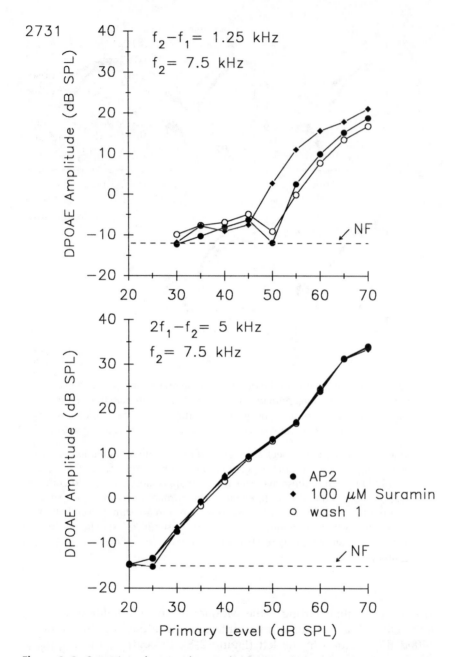

**Figure 2–8.** Suramin enhances the amplitude growth function for the quadratic ($f_2$–$f_1$) but not the cubic ($2f_1$–$f_2$) DPOAE. Shown are values obtained in a typical example following perfusion of the perilymph compartment with a second control artificial perilymph perfusion (AP2), suramin (100 $\mu$M), and a wash with AP (wash 1). The dashed line in each panel represents the average value of the noise floor.

diately after the silence period (Figure 2–9) with little effect on the overall shape of the change over time. Higher concentrations of PPADS (0.33 and 1 mM) induced a further suppression of the initial value and also reversed the decline, causing instead a slow dramatic rise (Figure 2–9). The subsequently recorded amplitude growth functions for the quadratic and cubic DPOAEs were shifted to the left (Figure 2–10).

Thus there are differences between the effects of these two ATP antagonists. Suramin appears to solely abolish the decline in the quadratic DPOAE whereas PPADS both (1) suppresses the initial, postsilence value of the DPOAE and (2) abolishes or reverses the decline. The reason for these differences in action of the two drugs is presently unknown; however, it may be the fact that PPADS is a more potent blocker of ATP than suramin. Both PPADS and suramin are equally potent in inhibiting ectonucleotidases (41% inhibition at 100 μM) (Ziganshin, Ziganshin, Bodin, Bailey, & Burnstock, 1995).

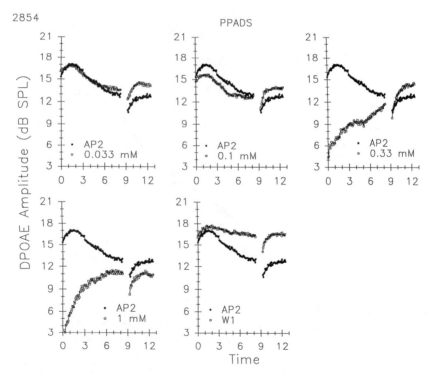

**Figure 2–9.** PPADS induces complex changes in the overall shape of the quadratic ($f_2$–$f_1$) DPOAE amplitude induced by continuous primary stimulation. Response amplitude as recorded following 15-min perfusions (in silence) of the perilymph compartment with the second artifical perilymph (AP2), increasing concentrations of PPADS (0.033–1.0 mM) and a wash with AP (wash). Data were collected as described in the legend for Figure 2–6.

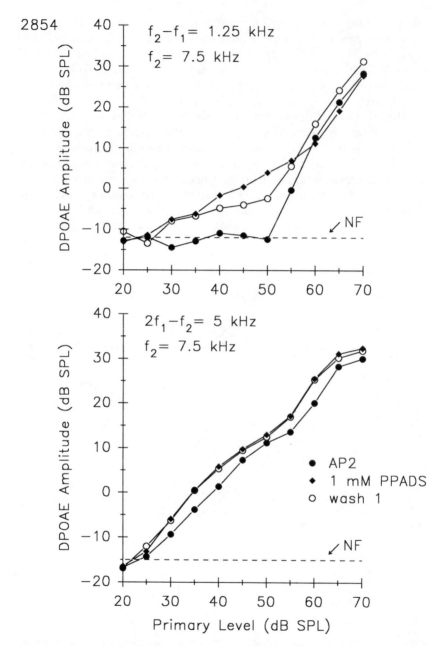

**Figure 2–10.** PPADS enhances the growth functions for the quadratic ($f_2$–$f_1$) and the cubic ($2f_1$–$f_2$) DPOAE. Shown are values obtained following collection of the data shown in Figure 2–9 for the second control perfusion (AP2), PPADS (1 mM), and a wash with AP. The dashed line in each panel represents the average value of the noise floor.

# ADDITIONAL CRITERIA

## Release Criterion (#3)

Evidence for the release criterion has been obtained from several sources. In the vestibular system, Bryant, Barron, Norris, & Guth (1987) demonstrated release of adenosine from the isolated semicircular canal in response to electrical stimulation. Because the authors made no attempt to block the degradation of any released ATP by ectonucleotidases, this adenosine may possibly represent an ATP breakdown product. If so, then Bryant et al. (1987) may well have demonstrated ATP release in response to depolarization of this hair cell containing organ.

Along similar lines, we have preliminary data to indicate that ATP release may be detected in effluent from the perilymph compartment. In an experiment carried out over 10 years ago with Drs. Bryant and Guth, increased levels of adenosine were detected in perilymph compartment effluent of guinea pig cochlea in response to raised potassium levels (see Bobbin in Bryant et al., 1987). Again this adenosine may represent an ATP breakdown product. This experiment may be taken as very preliminary evidence that ATP is released from cochlear tissue in response to depolarization and that it may be detected in perilymph effluent. The cells of origin of the adenosine (and therefore most probably the ATP) are unknown as the high potassium may have induced release from stria cells as well as inner hair cells, outer hair cells, Deiters' cells, and so forth. In addition, the potassium may have caused nonspecific swelling of the cells with the resultant spilling of the cytoplasmic ATP into the perilymph. Therefore these experiments will have to be replicated to determine if the adenosine (or ATP) release was calcium dependent and thus vesicular, and not due to cells leaking the contents of their cytoplasm.

Recently, Wangemann (1996) and Wangemann and Marcus (1994) demonstrated the calcium dependent release of ATP from isolated gerbil organ of Corti. The cellular source of the ATP is unknown. Likewise the resolution was not able to determine the target cells of the ATP that was released. The origin of the endogenous ATP that acts on the cells in the organ of Corti remains to be determined.

## Synthesis Criterion (#4)

The presence of isozymes of creatine kinase in Deiters' cells suggests that the released ATP may come from Deiters' cells (Spicer & Schulte, 1992). These enzymes synthesize ATP. Whether this ATP is the source of the ATP released onto the receptors on Deiters' cells surface to modulate the mechanics of the organ of Corti remains to be shown.

## Termination Criterion (#5)

Breakdown of any released ATP will be rapid as demonstrated by Vlajkovic, Thorne, Munoz, and Housley (1996), who presented evidence that ATP in perilymph is rapidly metabolized by ectonucleotidases to adenosine, adenosine 5'-diphosphate, and adenosine 5'-monophosphate. Therefore any released ATP will probably appear in perilymph effluent as one of these products. Thus the termination criterion (#5) appears to have been met, at least for ATP released into the perilymph compartment in the vicinity of the OHCs and Deiters' cells.

## Receptor Protein and mRNA Criterion (#6)

To date only a single P2X receptor type mRNA has been identified in the cochlea of rat (Brandle et al., 1997; Housley, Greenwood, Bennett, & Ryan, 1995). Guinea pig mRNA for P2X2 has also been found in an organ of Corti library (Parker, Bobbin, & Deininger, 1997). Thus the receptor protein and mRNA criterion (#6) is in the process of being met.

## SUMMARY AND MODEL

Currently, our model includes the endogenous release of ATP possibly from OHCs or Deiters' cells onto ATP receptors on Deiters' cells. This ATP may be released in response to a sound stimulus that depolarizes the OHC, inducing release of ATP from the OHC. Alternatively, sound may increase the concentration of potassium outside of Deiters' cells, inducing depolarization of Deiters' cells and subsequently the release of ATP from the Deiters' cells. The large concentration of the ATP synthesizing enzyme creatine kinase, in Deiters' cells, suggests that the source of exogenous ATP is the Deiters' cells. The released ATP will induce an influx of calcium (plus sodium) into the Deiters' cell through the ATP activated ion channel. This calcium may alter the mechanical stiffness of the Deiters' cell to increase or decrease the tension applied by the Deiters' cell on the OHCs. This in turn may adjust the cochlear amplifier in the face of a changing sound stimulus over time.

Based on the effects of the ATP antagonists, suramin and PPADS, we speculate that the continuous time varying amplitude change in the quadratic DPOAE may be a very sensitive measure of the effects of endogenous ATP acting in the above manner. We propose the following working model to explain the actions of the drugs. In this model, the magnitude of the quadratic DPOAE is determined by the amount of ATP acting at P2X2 receptors on Deiters' cells. The greater the amount of ATP acting on the receptors, then the larger this value. During silence, we propose that there is a basal level of ATP release. Upon turning on the primaries, the amount of ATP released is increased, producing the small increase in the quadratic

DPOAE seen at about 1 min into the primary stimulation. The subsequent decline in the quadratic DPOAE during continuous primary stimulation is then thought to be due to depletion of ATP from the release site. In addition, it is assumed that released ATP is rapidly broken down into inactive products by ectonucleotidases.

In this model, PPADS, a more powerful ATP antagonist than suramin, decreases the initial value of the quadratic DPOAE due to the block of ATP at receptors on Deiters' cells. The PPADS-induced inhibition of the ectonucleotidases (41% inhibition at 100 μM; Ziganshin, Ziganshin, Bodin, Bailey, & Burnstock, 1995) prevents the breakdown of ATP released in response to the presence of continuous primaries. The released ATP will accumulate in the extracellular space. This accumulated ATP will competitively displace PPADS from the receptors, allowing the ATP to act on the receptor. This receptor activation then reverses the decline in the quadratic DPOAE that occurs over time in the presence of continuous primaries.

In contrast, suramin is a weaker receptor antagonist, but equipotent with PPADS in inhibiting ectonucleotidases (41% inhibition at 100 μM) (Ziganshin et al., 1995). Any block of receptor by the suramin molecule is probably displaced by ATP accumulating in the extracellular space due to an inhibition of breakdown by the enzyme. Also, according to our single cell data, any accumulated ATP may be potentiated by suramin at the P2X2 receptor. This would explain the lack of effect of suramin on the initial value of the quadratic DPOAE. In addition, by blocking the breakdown of ATP, suramin would reverse the decline in the quadratic DPOAE.

This model does not take into consideration the possible location of metabotropic ATP receptors on OHCs, Deiters' cells, or Hensen's cells. The latter which are connected to Deiters' cells by gap junctions have ionotropic ATP receptors. In addition, many of the actions of the drugs that are described may be due to these other receptors. Therefore, the validity of this model will be determined by future research. However, the proposed model does explain the action of the drugs and allows for the design of further experiments.

**Acknowledgments:** The authors wish to thank Maureen Fallon for drawing the illustrations and Latasha Bright and Christopher LeBlanc for help. This work was supported in part by research grant numbers DC 00722-05 and DC00379 from the National Institute on Deafness and Other Communication Disorders, National Institutes of Health, and DAMD 17-93-V-3013, Kam's Fund for Hearing Research, and the Louisiana Lions Eye Foundation.

# REFERENCES

Ashmore, J. F., & Ohmori, H. (1990). Control of intracellular calcium by ATP in isolated outer hair cells of the guinea-pig cochlea. *Journal of Physiology, 428,* 109–131.

Aubert, A., Norris, C. H., & Guth, P. S. (1995). Indirect evidence for the presence and physiological role of endogenous extracellular ATP in the semicircular canal. *Neuroscience, 64,* 1153–1160.

Bledsoe, S. C., Jr., Bobbin, R. P., & Puel, J.-L. (1988). Neurotransmission in the inner ear. In A. F. Jahn & J. R. Santos-Sacchi (Eds.), *Physiology of hearing* (pp. 385–406). New York: Raven Press.

Bobbin, R. P. (1996). Chemical receptors on outer hair cells and their molecular mechanisms. In C. I. Berlin (Ed.), *Hair cells and hearing aids* (pp. 29–55). San Diego, CA: Singular Publishing Group.

Bobbin, R. P., Bledsoe, S. C., Jr., Winbery, S. L., & Jenison, G. L. (1985). Actions of putative neurotransmitters and other relevant compounds on *Xenopus* laevis lateral line. In D. G. Drescher (Ed.), *Auditory biochemistry* (pp. 102–122). Springfield, IL: Thomas.

Bobbin, R. P, Chen, C., Skellett, R. A., & Fallon, M. (1997). The ATP antagonist, suramin, prevents the time related decrease of the quadratic (f2–f1) otoacoustic distortion product. *Association for Research in Otolaryngology Abstracts, 54,* 14.

Bobbin, R. P., Chu, S. H. B., Skellett, R. A., Campbell, J., & Fallon, M. (1997). Cytotoxicity and mitogenicity of adenosine triphosphate in the cochlea. *Hearing Research, 113,* 155–164.

Bobbin, R. P., Fallon, M., Crist, J., Kujawa, S., & Erostegui, C. (1993). Intracochlear ATP reduces low intensity acoustic distortion products and CAP but does not change isolated OHC length. *Association for Research in Otolaryngology Abstracts, 16,* 102.

Bobbin, R. P., & Konishi, T. (1971a). Action of some cholinomimetics and cholinolytics on the effect of the crossed olivocochlear bundle (COCB). *Journal of the Acoustical Society of America, 49,* 122.

Bobbin, R. P., & Konishi, T. (1971b). Acetylcholine mimics crossed olivocochlear bundle stimulation. *Nature New Biology, 231,* 222–223.

Bobbin, R. P., & Konishi, T. (1974). Action of cholinergic and anticholinergic drugs at the crossed olivocochlear bundle-hair cell junction. *Acta Oto-laryngologica (Oslo), 77,* 56–65.

Bobbin, R. P., Morgan, D. N., & Bledsoe, S. C., Jr. (1979). Action of glutamate and related substances on the spontaneous activity of afferent nerves in the toad lateral line. *Society of Neuroscience Abstracts, 5,* 16.

Bobbin, R. P., & Thompson, M. H. (1978). Effects of putative transmitters on afferent cochlear transmission. *Annals of Otology, Rhinology, and Laryngology, 87,* 185–190.

Brandle, U., Spielmanns, P., Osteroth, R., Sim, J., Surprenant, A., Buell, G., Ruppersberg, J. P., Plinkert, P. K., Zenner, H. P., & Glowatzki, E. (1997). Desensitization of the $P2x_2$ receptor controlled by alternative splicing. *FEBS Letters (Amsterdam), 404,* 294–298.

Brown, A. M. (1988). Continuous low level sound alters cochlear mechanics: An efferent effect? *Hearing Research, 34,* 27–38.

Brownell, W. E. (1996). Outer hair cell electromotility and otoacoustic emissions. In C. I. Berlin (Ed.), *Hair cells and hearing aids* (pp. 3–28). San Diego, CA: Singular Publishing Group.

Bryant, G. M., Barron, S. E., Norris, C. H., & Guth, P. S. (1987). Adenosine is a modulator of hair cell-afferent neurotransmission. *Hearing Research, 30,* 231–237.

Burnstock, G. (1990). Purinergic mechanisms. In G. R. Dubyak & J. S. Fedan (Eds.), *Biological Actions of Extracellular ATP. Annals of New York Acadamy of Science, 603,* 1–18.

Chen, C., LeBlanc, C., & Bobbin, R. P. (1997). Differences in the distribution of responses to ATP and acetylcholine between outer hair cells of rat and guinea pig. *Hearing Research, 110,* 87–94.

Chen, C., Nenov, A., & Bobbin, R. P. (1995). Noise exposure alters the response of outer hair cells to ATP. *Hearing Research, 88,* 215–221.

Chen, C., Nenov, A. P., Norris, C., & Bobbin, R. P. (1995). ATP modulation of L-type $Ca^{2+}$ channel currents in guinea pig outer hair cells. *Hearing Research, 86,* 25–33.

Chu, S. H. B., Fallon, M., Skellett, R. A., Campbell, J., LeBlanc, C. S., & Bobbin, R. P. (1997). Adenosine triphosphate (ATP) induces outer hair cell death. *Association for Research in Otolaryngology Abstracts, 294,* 74.

Collo, G., North, R. A., Kawashima, E., Merlo-Pich, E., Neidhart, S., Surprenant, A., & Buell, G. (1996). Cloning of $P2X_5$ and $P2X_{6x}$ receptors and the distribution and properties of an extended family of ATP-gated ion channels. *Journal of Neuroscience, 16,* 2495–2507.

Dulon, D. (1995). $Ca^{2+}$ signaling in Deiters cells of the guinea-pig cochlea active process in supporting cells? In A. Flock, D. Ottoson, & M. Ulfendahl (Eds.), *Active hearing* (pp. 195–207). Great Britain: Elsevier Science Ltd.

Dulon, D., Blanchet, C., & Laffon, E. (1994). Photo-released intracellular $Ca^{2+}$ evokes reversible mechanical responses in supporting cells of the guinea-pig organ of Corti. *Biochemical and Biophysical Research Communications, 201,* 1263–1269.

Dulon, D., Moataz, R., & Mollard, P. (1993). Characterization of $Ca^{2+}$ signals generated by extracellular nucleotides in supporting cells of the organ of Corti. *Cell Calcium, 14,* 245–254.

Dulon, D., Mollard, P., & Aran, J.-M. (1991). Extracellular ATP elevates cytosolic $Ca^{2+}$ in cochlear inner hair cells. *NeuroReport, 2,* 69–72.

Eybalin, M. (1993). Neurotransmitters and neuromodulators of the mammalian cochlea. *Physiological Reviews, 73,* 309–373.

Frank, G., & Kossl, M. (1996). The acoustic two-tone distortions $2f_1$–$f_2$ and $f_2$–$f_1$ and their possible relation to changes in the operating point of the cochlear amplifier. *Hearing Research, 98,* 104–115.

Housley, G. D., Greenwood, D., & Ashmore, J. F. (1992). Localization of cholinergic and purinergic receptors on outer hair cells isolated from the guinea-pig cochlea. *Proceedings of the Royal Society of London, Series B: Biological Sciences (London), 249,* 265–273.

Housley, G. D., Greenwood, D., Bennett, T., & Ryan, A. F. (1995). Identification of a short form of the P2xR1-purinoceptor subunit produced by alternative splicing in the pituitary and cochlea. *Biochemical and Biophysical Research Communications, 212,* 501–508.

Ikeda, K., Saito, Y., Nishiyama, A., & Takasaka, T. (1991). Effect of neuroregulators on the intracellular calcium level in the outer hair cell isolated from the guinea pig. *Otology, Rhinology, and Laryngology, 53,* 78–81.

Kakehata, S., Nakagawa, T., Takasaka, T., & Akaike, N. (1993). Cellular mechanism of acetylcholine-induced response in dissociated outer hair cells of guinea-pig cochlea. *Journal of Physiology, 463,* 227–244.

Kirk, D. L., & Johnstone, B. M. (1993). Modulation of $f_2$–$f_1$: Evidence for a GABA-ergic efferent system in apical cochlea of the guinea pig. *Hearing Research, 67,* 20–34.

Kujawa, S. G., Erostegui, C., Fallon, M., Crist, J., & Bobbin, R. P. (1994). Effects of adenosine 5'-triphosphate and related agonists on cochlear function. *Hearing Research, 76,* 87–100.

Kujawa, S. G., Fallon, M., & Bobbin, R. P. (1993). Alterations in cochlear electrical potentials by intracochlear ATP and analogs. *Society of Neuroscience Abstracts, 19,* 1419.

Kujawa, S. G., Fallon, M., & Bobbin, R. P. (1994). ATP antagonists cibacron blue, basilen blue and suramin alter sound-evoked responses of the cochlea and auditory nerve. *Hearing Research, 78,* 181–188.

Kujawa, S. G., Fallon, M., & Bobbin, R. P. (1995). Time-varying alterations in the $f_2$–$f_1$ DPOAE response to continuous primary stimulation. I. Response characterization and contribution of the olivocochlear efferents. *Hearing Research, 85,* 142–154.

Kujawa, S. G., Fallon, M., Skellett, R. A., & Bobbin, R. P. (1996). Time-varying alterations in the $f_2$–$f_1$ DPOAE response to continuous primary stimulation. II. Influence of local calcium-dependent mechanisms. *Hearing Research, 97,* 153–164.

Liu, J., Kozakura, K., & Marcus, D. C. (1995). Evidence for purinergic receptors in vestibular dark cell and strial marginal cell epithelia of the gerbil. *Auditory Neuroscience, 1,* 331–340.

Lowe, M., & Robertson, D. (1995). The behaviour of the $f_2$–$f_1$ acoustic distortion product: Lack of effect of brainstem lesions in anaesthetized guinea pigs. *Hearing Research, 83,* 133–141.

Mockett, B. G., Bo, X., Housley, G. D., Thorne, P. R., & Burnstock, G. (1995). Autoradiographic labelling of P2 purinoceptors in the guinea-pig cochlea. *Hearing Research, 84,* 177–193.

Mockett, B. G., Housley, G. D., & Thorne, P. R. (1994). Fluorescence imaging of extracellular purinergic receptor sites and putative ecto-ATPase sites on isolated cochlear hair cells. *Journal of Neuroscience, 14,* 6992–7007.

Mroz, E. A., & Sewell, W. F. (1989). Pharmacological alterations of the activity of afferent fibers innervating hair cells. *Hearing Research, 38,* 11–162.

Munoz, D. J. B., Thorne, P. R., Housley, G. D., & Billett, T. E. (1995). Adenosine 5'-triphosphate (ATP) concentrations in the endolymph and perilymph of the guinea pig cochlea. *Hearing Research, 90,* 119–125.

Munoz, D. J. B., Thorne, P. R., Housley, G. D., Billett, T. E., & Battersby, J. M. (1995). Extracellular adenosine 5'-triphosphate (ATP) in the endolymphatic compartment influences cochlear function. *Hearing Research, 90,* 106–118.

Nakagawa, T., Akaike, N., Kimitsuki, T., Komune, S., & Arima, T. (1990). ATP-induced current in isolated outer hair cells of guinea pig cochlea. *Journal of Neurophysiology, 63,* 1068–1074.

Parker, M. S., Bobbin, R. P., & Deininger, P. L. (1997). Guinea pig organ of Corti contains mRNA for ATP receptor type P2x2. *Association for Research in Otolaryngology Abstracts, 20,* 217.

Shigemoto, T., & Ohmori, H. (1990). Muscarinic agonists and ATP increase the intracellular $Ca^{2+}$ concentration in chick cochlear hair cells. *Journal of Physiology, 420,* 127–148.

Skellett, R. A., Chen, C., Fallon, M., Nenov, A. P., & Bobbin, R. P. (1997). Pharmacological evidence that endogenous ATP modulates cochlear mechanics. *Hearing Research, 111*, 42–54.

Spicer, S. S., & Schulte, B. A. (1992). Creatine kinase in epithelium of the inner ear. *Journal of Histochemistry and Cytochemistry, 40*, 185–192.

Sugasawa, M., Erostegui, C., Blanchet, C., & Dulon, D. (1996). ATP activates non-selective cation channels and calcium release in inner hair cells of the guinea-pig cochlea. *Journal of Physiology, 491.3*, 707–718.

Suzuki, M., Ikeda, K., Sunose, H., Hozawa, K., Kusakari, C., Katori, Y., & Takasaka, T. (1995). ATP-induced increase in intracellular $Ca^{2+}$ concentration in the cultured marginal cell of the stria vascularis of guinea-pigs. *Hearing Research, 86*, 68–76.

Vlajkovic, S. M., Thorne, P. R., Munoz, D. J. B., & Housley, G. D. (1996). Ectonucleotidase activity in the perilymphatic compartment of the guinea pig cochlea. *Hearing Research, 99*, 31–37.

Wang, D., Huang, N., Heller, E. J., & Heppel, L. A. (1994). A novel synergistic stimulation of Swiss 3T3 cells by extracellular ATP and mitogens with opposite effects on cAMP levels. *Journal of Biological Chemistry, 269*, 16648–16655.

Wangemann, P. (1995). Comparison of ion transport mechanisms between vestibular dark cells and strial marginal cells. *Hearing Research, 90*, 149–157.

Wangemann, P. (1996). $Ca^{2+}$ dependent release of ATP from the organ of Corti measured with a luciferin-lucerferase bioluminescence assay. *Auditory Neuroscience, 2*, 187–192.

Wangemann, P., & Marcus, D. C. (1994). K+-induced ATP release from the organ of Corti from the inner ear measured with the luciferin-luciferase bioluminescence assay in vitro. *Society of Neuroscience Abstracts, 20*, 1276.

White, P. N., Thorne, P. R., Housley, G. D., Mockett, B., Billett, T. E., & Burnstock, G. (1995). Quinacrine staining of marginal cells in the stria vascularis of the guinea-pig cochlea: A possible source of extracellular ATP? *Hearing Research, 90*, 97–105.

Ziganshin, A. U., Ziganshin, L. E., Bodin, P., Bailey, D., & Burnstock, G. (1995). Effects of P2-purinoceptor antagonists on ecto-nucleotidase activity of guinea-pig vas deferens cultured smooth muscle cells. *Biochemistry and Molecular Biology International, 36*, 863–869.

Zoeteweij, J. P., Van de Water, B., De Bont, H. J. G. M., & Nagelkerke, J. F. (1996). The role of a purinergic $P_{2z}$ receptor in calcium-dependent cell killing of isolated rat hepatocytes by extracellular adenosine triphosphate. *Hepatology, 23*, 858–865.

# 3

# Origin and Implications of Two "Components" in Distortion Product Otoacoustic Emissions

*David M. Mills, Ph.D.*
Virginia Merrill Bloedel Hearing Research Center
Department of Otolaryngology, Head and Neck Surgery
University of Washington
Seattle, Washington

Distortion product otoacoustic emissions have proven very useful in both clinical and laboratory settings as noninvasive indicators of cochlear functioning (e.g., Rübsamen, Mills, & Rubel, 1995; review: Probst, Lonsbury-Martin, & Martin, 1991). However, there remain several puzzling, anomalous, and apparently disparate phenomena which threaten to limit their usefulness.

The appearance of "notches" in input-output or "growth" functions has been noted in both emission and psychoacoustic studies of the cubic distortion tone (e.g., Brown, 1987; Smoorenburg, 1972; Whitehead, Lonsbury-Martin, & Martin, 1992a, 1992b). The notch in emission is revealed when, as the stimulus amplitude is increased, the emission amplitude decreases suddenly and then recovers. The phase of the emission usually changes rapidly as the notch region is traversed. The notches typically occur once in a growth function, at moderate stimulus levels, although they may not be observed at all for some parameter choices. The existence of such regions of rapid amplitude and phase changes complicates certain measurements. For example, measurements of group delay, which depend on phase angle measurements, must avoid such regions to avoid anomalous results (Brown & Kemp, 1985).

The contribution of apparent "passive" emissions from the cochlea also leads to problems with measurement. In terms of absolute levels, only emission measurements at low stimulus levels have been considered good indicators of cochlear function (e.g., Brown, McDowell, & Forge, 1989; Rübsamen et al., 1995). Emissions at very high stimulus levels usually are only moderately dependent on the quality of cochlear function and even continue after the death of an animal (Schmiedt & Adams, 1981). It has generally been assumed that these emissions do not give a useful indication of cochlear function. Nonetheless, these high level emissions have been shown to be of cochlear origin. Their comparative insensitivity has led to the suggestion that it is appropriate to categorize emissions as "active" or "passive" to indicate their probable origins (Brown, 1987; Brown et al., 1989; Johnstone, Gleich, Mavadat, McAlpine, & Kapadia, 1990; Lonsbury-Martin, Martin, Probst, & Coats, 1987; Mills, Norton, & Rubel, 1994; Mills & Rubel, 1994; Norton, Bargones, & Rubel, 1991; Whitehead et al., 1992a, 1992b). This suggestion remains controversial, and, further, it is difficult to know how to conceptualize the origin of emissions at *moderate* stimulus levels. These emissions are clearly affected by cochlear functioning, but their behavior is acutely dependent on stimulus parameters. For example, the emission amplitude for moderate stimulus levels may *increase* sharply immediately after the death of the animal, or may decrease or change little for similar parameters (Mills & Rubel, 1994).

Although the "notch" is not always obvious on a given choice of parameters for an input-output function, it is noteworthy that when it is apparent, it occurs at the moderate stimulus levels characteristic of these confusing, neither "active" nor "passive," responses. The notch therefore seems to divide the growth function broadly into an "active" and a "passive" region.

Earlier experiments comparing living to dead cochleas have been supplemented by more selective manipulations, such as temporary anoxia and acute diuretic effects (Kemp & Brown, 1984; Mills et al., 1993; Mills & Rubel, 1994; Rebillard & Lavigne-Rebillard, 1992; Rübsamen et al., 1995; Whitehead et al., 1992b). Both methods cause a rapid and reversible lowering of the endocochlear potential (EP). As the EP decreases, there is a progressive impairment of cochlear amplifier function. The experiments provide a model system for studying the cochlear amplifier function with varying degrees of impairment. Typically, emissions for low stimulus levels drop relatively rapidly to the noise floor, whereas those at high stimulus levels decrease slowly and modestly. Emissions for moderate stimulus levels typically drop rapidly, but then hit a sharp minimum, and recover quickly but partially to a relatively unchanging emission level. It is tempting to identify the relatively unchanging emission found during the maximal effect of the diuretic as the "passive" response, and we have done so (e.g., Mills et al., 1994; Mills & Rubel, 1996). All the more tempting, as these points at the maximal diuretic effect usually lie on a growth function that is straight and without a notch. The slope of the growth function is, however, about two. If the animal is euthanized, the emissions at moderate stimulus levels decrease still further. The slope of the growth function found postmortem is more typically three, as would be expected for truly passive emissions. Should it be concluded that there are *two* "passive" kinds of emissions?

Recently, there have been a series of experiments using emissions as a sensitive assay to detect the effects of efferent functioning (Kujawa & Liberman, 1996; Liberman, Puria, & Guinan, 1996; Puel & Rebillard, 1990; Williams & Brown, 1995). The effects on the emissions depend strongly on the choice of emission parameters, and the same intervention can cause a sharp decrease or increase in the emission amplitude. It is noteworthy that the most extreme results seem to be obtained when the parameters are near a notch in the growth function. Because the origin of the extreme variability in emission response is not known, it seems difficult to know how to interpret experiments of these kinds in the absence of a model.

## EMISSION MODEL

A very simple, pragmatic emission model appears adequate to provide explanations for most of these phenomena. There are two necessary and independent assumptions: (1) Saturation of the gain of the cochlear amplifier is the major source of nonlinearity in the cochlea. (2) Emissions from different regions of the cochlea will not necessarily sum in phase. These assumptions will be elaborated in turn. Additional details may be found in Mills (1997).

At sufficiently low signal levels the response of the cochlea must be linear, although this range may actually lie below the threshold for a neural response (Nuttall & Dolan, 1996). That is, at very low stimulus levels, the cochlear response to two or more sinusoidal stimuli (i.e., frequencies $f_1$, $f_1$, . . . ) would be the algebraic sum of the response to either alone. The gain of the cochlear amplifier, however, is limited. As stimulus levels increase, eventually the gain at any one frequency will be reduced by the presence of other signals, as well as by the amplitude of the traveling wave at this frequency. To proceed, the very simple assumption is made that the instantaneous gain at any point depends on the instantaneous amplitude of all the signals present at that point. It is also assumed that the traveling waves interact *only* through this gain reduction, so that the quasilinear approximation continues to be useful. That is, the total cochlear response can be assumed to be approximately made up of the sum of separate traveling waves, each having its own frequency.

The specific form of the reduction in instantaneous gain is chosen to be compatible with the form of the saturation in outer hair cell input-output functions, as well as many other biologically relevant systems, that is, a Boltzman or hyberbolic tangent function. Such a function gives a relatively sharp reduction in gain as the instantaneous amplitude increases past a characteristic level, the "saturation level." However, note that the instantaneous amplitude of the cochlear response is generally given by the sum of sinusoidal signals of different frequencies. Even if the peak response of this sum is well into saturation, there are still portions of the cycle near the zero crossings where the response amplitude is quite low. Gain would still be available to amplify the traveling wave at these moments. The amount of gain available on average is approximately proportional to the inverse of the total peak amplitude of the cochlear response at that point. This is approximately the proportion of time that the total signal is near a zero crossing.

A simple analogy for this situation is pushing a swing. When the amplitude of the motion is low, one can add energy through the whole cycle. When the amplitude of the motion is high, one wisely attempts to apply force only near the times of zero velocity.

The results of a precise calculation of the effect of saturation on the average cochlear amplifier gain at any location are given in Figure 3–1. As noted, the effect of saturation is to introduce a scale factor, the "saturation level." By our normalization, the average cochlear amplifier gain is reduced to 75% of its normal value when the peak cochlear response amplitude is equal to the saturation level. For simplicity, this saturation level will be assumed to be independent of frequency and position in the cochlea. In what follows, all cochlear response amplitudes will be given in terms of this level.

As noted before, when the amplitude of the total cochlear resonse at any point is much greater than the saturation level, the gain reduction is approximately proportional to the inverse of the scaled cochlear response. That is, if the cochlear response were three times the saturation level, the cochlear amplifier gain at that point would be reduced to approximately one third of its normal value. For example, if the rate of amplification were 30 dB/mm along the cochlea at low levels, it would be reduced to 10 dB/mm when the cochlear response amplitude was three times the saturation level. This point is identified on Figure 3–1 for comparison with the exact response. It can be seen that the approximation is quite good for this and all higher response amplitudes. In logarithmic units, the approximation is thus adequate whenever the total cochlear response is 10 dB or more above the saturation level.

The effect of the saturation on the cochlear response for a single tone stimulus is summarized in Figure 3–2. The horizontal axis gives the distance along the basilar membrane (BM) from the base of the cochlea. The distance is expressed in octave units, meaning that the location is identified by the frequency at which a low amplitude stimulus will produce the max-

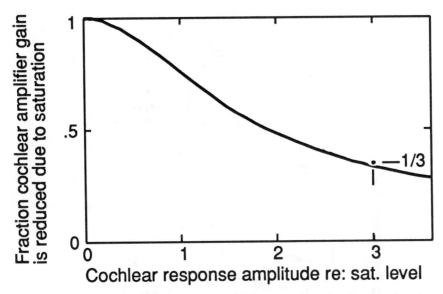

**Figure 3–1.** The assumed reduction in gain due to signal amplitude at any location in the cochlea. To use this relationship to calculate the cochlear amplifier gain, the total amplitude of all signals present at that location is computed and the point is located on the horizontal axis. The appropriate amplitude for this case is the linear sum of the peak amplitudes (over the cycle) present at each frequency. Note that the horizontal scale is linear (not logarithmic) amplitude and that it is normalized to the characteristic saturation level. The vertical axis then gives the reduction in gain for any traveling wave which is in its active amplification zone. The fraction reduction is the average reduction over the cycle and multiplies the base cochlear amplification rate (expressed in dB/octave or dB/mm).

imum response. The frequency of the tone shown has been chosen to be two octaves below the base frequency, so that the maximum response (at low stimulus levels) occurs at the position denoted z = 2. The stimulus for the lowest curve is 100 dB below the saturation level. As this wave travels from the base, there is first a modest increase in amplitude due to passive mechanical characteristics. At approximately the location where the passive response would peak, the cochlear amplifier begins to amplify the traveling wave. The rate of amplification shown is 100 dB/octave. In slightly over a half octave, the cochlear response reaches its peak as losses begin to dominate. There is then a very rapid decline following this peak as the wave energy dissipates. At these low stimulus levels, there is a total increase in amplitude of 60 dB for the model parameters chosen.

There are three other responses shown in Figure 3–2, all for the same frequency but for stimulus levels successively 40 dB higher (i.e., 100 times). As the stimulus level is increased, the effects of saturation in reducing the

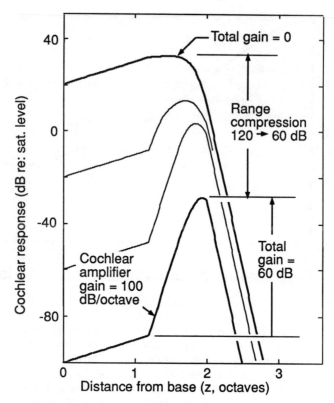

**Figure 3–2.** Cochlear response for single tone stimuli, showing curves for four different stimulus levels at the same frequency. The horizontal axis gives the distance along the basilar membrane as distance from the base in octaves. Note that the frequency decreases with distance from the base, so the frequency shown is two octaves below the base cutoff frequency. The basic cochlear amplifier gain is 100 dB/octave for all four levels. For stimuli 100 dB below the saturation level, this amplification rate leads to a total gain of 60 dB. This is the improvement in peak response at this stimulus level with a functioning cochlear amplifier compared to none. As the stimulus level is increased, saturation effects at the higher amplitudes progressively reduce the gain, until there is no detectable gain for a stimulus level 20 dB above the saturation level.

cochlear amplifier gain become more apparent. For a stimulus level 20 dB above the saturation level, the cochlear amplifier gain is approximately zero throughout, and the response becomes essentially passive. Note that the range of the peak cochlear response would be 120 dB over these four stimulus levels if the cochlear amplifier were not functional. In contrast, as noted in Figure 3–2, the range is only 60 dB when it is functioning.

The model is constructed so that it is quite easy to extend calculations from a single stimulus at one frequency to several different stimuli at several different frequencies. For each stimulus frequency, the gain in its active amplification zone is reduced according to Figure 3–1. The cochlear response amplitude used in the calculation is just the (linear) sum of the amplitudes of all the waves present at that point along the basilar membrane. Typical results of such calculations are shown in Figure 3–3. Each panel represents the cochlear response for a different stimulus level. The top panel summarizes the cochlear response with a stimulus level 20 dB above the saturation level, and the bottom panel shows the response for a stimulus level 100 dB below the saturation level. Each panel illustrates the cochlear traveling wave amplitude along the basilar membrane. The response at $f_1$ is indicated by a dashed line, the response at $f_2$ by a light solid line, and the emission generated at each point at the frequency $2f_1-f_2$ by a heavy solid line. The horizontal axis is the distance from the base, measured in octaves, and is a linear scale. That is, the number of millimeters per octave is assumed constant along the cochlear duct. The vertical axis indicates response amplitude and is a logarithmic scale, given in dB.

The emission generated at any point was calculated from the following formula. For small signal amplitudes, from a power series approximation it can be shown that emission generated at the frequency $(mf_1 \pm nf_2)$ is approximately proportional to $(y_1)^m(y_2)^n$, where $y_1$ and $y_2$ are the instantaneous cochlear response amplitudes at frequencies $f_1$ and $f_2$, and m and n are any positive integers. The approximation is appropriate for all physiologically relevant functions, i.e., for functions in which there are not discontinuities at or near the operating point. The use of this approximation also requires the quasilinear assumption to remain valid. The approximation will be expected to fail at high stimulus levels where the approximation will predict higher emission amplitudes than a more complete analysis would estimate. That is, the actual emission amplitudes, and those from a more complete model, must saturate at high enough stimulus levels. At the least, the amplitude cannot continue to rise as a high power of the signal amplitude.

To calculate the total emission amplitude seen in the ear canal, the emission distribution shown in Figure 3–3 must be integrated over the length of the cochlea. However, the approximation gives only the amplitude of the emission. The emission generated at each point also has an associated phase angle, which depends on the stimulus phases at the point of generation. As the emissions travel back along the basilar membrane toward the ear canal, they suffer phase rotations, the amount depending on their point of origin. More significantly, the phases of the forward traveling waves begin to change rapidly as their peaks are reached. The phase angle

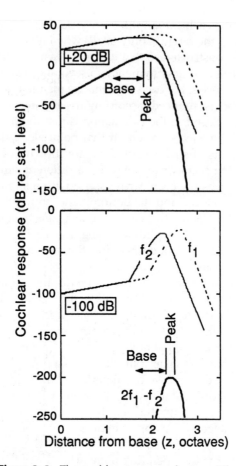

**Figure 3–3.** The cochlear response for two different stimuli present simultaneously. The stimuli are of equal amplitude and their frequency ratio is $f_2/f_1$ = 1.28. In the upper panel, the stimulus levels are both 20 dB above the saturation level, while the levels are 100 dB below the saturation level in the lower panel. The peak amplitude of the traveling wave at the frequency $f_1$ is shown by the light dashed line, and that at $f_2$ by the light solid line. The emission generated at the frequency $2f_1-f_2$ is indicated by the heavy solid line. Note that this is the generation rate for the emission, not the traveling wave at this frequency. To obtain the amplitude of the reverse traveling wave the emission generated must be integrated over the length of the cochlea. In this model, it is assumed that the major non-zero emission contributions originate in the two regions indicated "base" and "peak."

is important because emissions summing with phases 180 degrees different will tend to cancel each other.

A simplifying assumption is needed. With guidance from phase measurements along the cochlea (e.g., Robles, Ruggero, & Rich, 1986), it is assumed that the emission generation can be divided into three regions. First, there is assumed to be a (large) region basal to the location of the peak of the emission in which the phase angle changes from all effects are small. The emission from this whole "base" region will be assumed to sum in phase. The edge of this region is necessarily defined when the emission angle starts changing rapidly as the distance along the BM increases. The boundary could be defined, for example, as the point at which the phase angle becomes 90 degrees to the previous sum. Following this boundary will be a region where the emission phase goes from 90 degrees to 270 degrees, presumably fairly rapidly, and the summed emission from this necessarily small region will be on average 180 degrees to that from the first region. The emission phases in the third region, apical to the second region, are assumed to vary so rapidly that they contribute nothing to the total emission.

For concreteness in the calculation, it is now assumed that the second region is a small region centered on the emission peak, of size only about one eighth octave. This is the most tentative of all the assumptions in this simple model. It can be justified at this point primarily by the useful results this assumption produces and the agreement with observation. The two regions, "base" and "peak," which contribute to the total emission are indicated in Figure 3–3. Note that the relative contributions of the two regions are not immediately obvious from Figure 3–3, because of the logarithmic display used for the amplitudes. However, an exact calculation supports what might be suspected from the distributions shown. At low stimulus levels, the majority of the emissions come from the region of the sharp peak. At high stimulus levels, the majority come from the broad, base region.

## MODEL RESULTS

The emission model characterized previously produces the emission patterns along the BM at $2f_1-f_2$ illustrated in Figure 3–3. Integrating the emission distribution according to the previous discussion produces the net emission shown in Figure 3–4, as a function of stimulus amplitude. The stimulus amplitudes at $f_1$ and $f_2$ are assumed to be equal ($L_1 = L_2$) with a moderate frequency ratio ($f_2/f_1 = 1.28$) typical of many experimental designs. The stimulus level (on the horizontal axis) extends from 100 dB below the saturation level to equal to it. The growth functions are presented over this range for cochlear amplifier gains from 0 to 100 dB/octave.

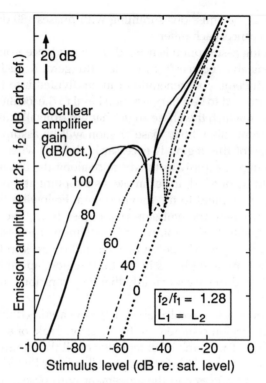

**Figure 3–4.** Input-output or "growth" functions from the model for the emission at $2f_1-f_2$. Equal stimulus levels are assumed ($L_1 = L_2$) and the frequency ratio is $f_2/f_1 = 1.28$. The emission (on the vertical axis) is calculated for stimulus levels from 100 dB below the saturation level to a stimulus level equal to the saturation level (on the horizontal axis). The parameter gives the basic cochlear amplifier gain for each calculation. Note the sharp notch found in nearly all the responses near 40–45 dB below the saturation level.

The following general results may be noted. At both high and low stimulus levels, the $2f_1-f_2$ emission varies as the third power of the stimulus level. This is expected from the simple approximation employed for their calculation, of course. At low stimulus levels, however, the emission is sharply peaked and the majority of emission comes from the peak region indicated in Figure 3–3. At high stimulus levels, the emission distribution is quite broad and therefore the base region contributes the majority of the summed emission. At some intermediate level, the emission from these two regions must be equal and the total emission will sum to zero. On a logarithmic plot, this zero causes a sharp notch, as shown in Figure 3–4. The stimulus level where the notch occurs changes slightly and in a complex manner as the cochlear amplifier gain is changed. However, the position is relatively stable, and is typically located at stimulus levels 40–45 dB below the saturation level, for the parameter choices in Figure 3–3.

Experiments that decrease the endocochlear potential sharply can be considered experiments in which the cochlear amplifier gain is decreased. This is a system for investigating the effect of changing the cochlear amplifier gain over the range from normal to zero. Therefore, it is useful to examine the appearance of the emissions observed when the stimulus level is kept constant but the cochlear amplifier gain is varied. Such responses are illustrated in Figure 3–5 for the same parameters as in Figure 3–4.

There are three different characteristic results depending on the stimulus level. For high stimulus levels, that is, those seen at the top of Figure 3–5B which are near the saturation level, the emission amplitude decreases slowly and monotonically as the cochlear amplifier gain decreases. For the whole range of cochlear amplifier gain from 100 dB/octave to zero, the decrease in the emission amplitude is only about 10 dB. The opposite effect is found with small stimulus amplitudes, shown at the bottom of this panel. With a stimulus level about 70 dB below the saturation level, or lower, the emission drops rapidly to the noise floor as the cochlear amplifier gain decreases. Again, the decrease in the observable range is monotonic with the cochlear amplifier gain.

In contrast, for stimulus levels near where the "notch" in Figure 3–4 is seen, that is, near 40–50 dB below the saturation level, there is quite complex behavior. Consider the response for a stimulus level 50 dB below the saturation level. As the cochlear amplifier gain first begins to decrease from 100 dB/octave, the emission amplitude actually *increases* slightly. Near 80 dB/octave it reaches a maximum and then declines slowly. The emission amplitude then plunges to a sharp minimum at a cochlear amplifier gain of about 35 dB/octave and then rebounds. There is another broad maximum and then a gradual decrease to reach a finite value at zero gain.

The change in phase angle for typical responses is summarized in Figure 3–5A. For high level stimuli, the phase angle never changes. However, the phase for lower level stimuli begins 180 degrees different than that for high level stimuli. When the zero (notch) is passed, the phase angle rapidly changes by 180 degrees to match the high amplitude phase angle.

All of the behaviors illustrated in Figure 3–5 have been observed, although certainly not well understood previously (Mills et al., 1993; Mills & Rubel, 1994, 1996). The advantage of such a model is that the origins of this complex behavior can be explored in detail. Such an exploration is summarized in Figure 3–6.

All of the responses in Figure 3–6 are for the same stimulus level, 50 dB below the saturation level. In each row, the results for one cochlear

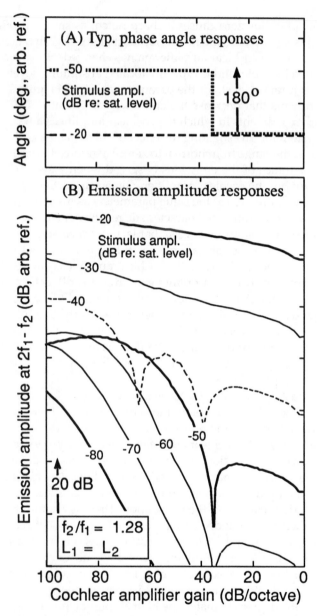

**Figure 3–5.** The figure covers the same parameter ranges as Figure 3–4, but instead of displaying curves for varying stimulus level with cochlear amplifier gain as a parameter, here the cochlear amplifier gain is varied and the stimulus level is the parameter. Both panels indicate the behavior of the $2f_1-f_2$ distortion product but (A) displays the phase angle response whereas (B) gives the amplitude responses for different stimulus levels.

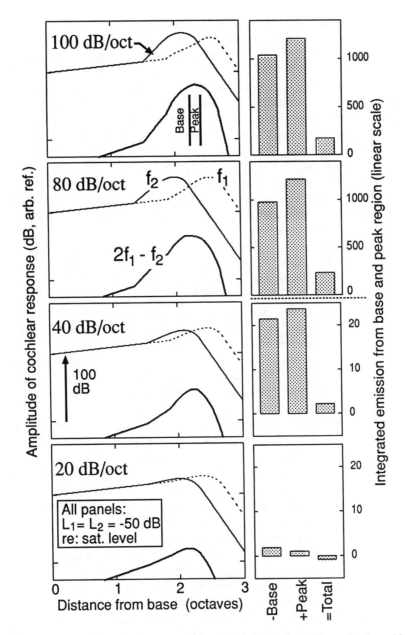

**Figure 3–6.** The left panels illustrate cochlear responses for four different basic cochlear amplifier gain conditions but the same stimulus level. The same conventions are employed as in Figure 3–3. The right panels show the result of integrating the emission generation over the "base" and "peak" areas indicated in the top left panel. Note that the vertical scale on the left panels is logarithmic, whereas it is linear on the right panels. For all panels, the stimulus levels are equal to 50 dB below the saturation level. The frequency ratio is $f_2/f_1 = 1.28$.

amplifier gain are presented. For example, the top row summarizes results for the case with the cochlear amplifier gain of 100 dB/octave. In the left panel, the response along the length of the cochlea is summarized using the same conventions as Figure 3–3. That is, the response at $f_1$ is shown by a dashed line, at $f_2$ by a light solid line, and the resulting emission generation at $2f_1-f_2$ by a heavy solid line. The amplitude scale is logarithmic and given in dB, whereas the distance scale is linear and given in octaves from the base. The right panel summarizes the results of summing the emissions in the two areas separately, and then combining them assuming they are 180 degrees out of phase. Note that the right panel ordinates are linear, with the same (arbitrary) scale factor used throughout. The sign convention is that emissions from the peak are positive and those from the base are negative. Note that there is change in the displayed scale between the top two panels and the bottom two panels.

The message here is simple: For this particular stimulus level, as the cochlear amplifier gain changes, the emission from the two regions is always nearly the same, and so nearly cancels to zero. This simple fact explains all of the complex behavior noted in Figure 3–5. First, consider the case at the start when the gain is 100 dB/octave. The emission from the peak region is slightly larger than that from the base, so that the net emission, which is much smaller in magnitude, comes from the peak. However, the high gain causes significant saturation at this stimulus level, resulting in modestly broad peaks in the cochlear responses. At a gain of 100 dB/octave, there are relatively high base emissions compared to that for a cochlear amplifier gain 20 dB/octave lower, shown on the panels on the next row down. When the gain decreases to 80 dB/octave, the traveling wave amplitudes become smaller and the emission from both the base and peak region decreases. However, because the saturation decreases, the peak response itself is almost as high as at larger gain. The emission from the peak region decreases slightly less than that from the base, leading to a modest *increase* in the difference. This accounts for the increase in emission of a few dB seen in Figure 3–5, as the gain decreases from 100 to 80 dB/octave.

The lower two panels illustrate the changes that occur as the notch area is traversed. At a cochlear amplifier gain of 40 dB/octave, the emission from the peak still is slightly larger than that from the base. However, at gains of 20 dB/octave, the base emission now slightly exceeds the peak emission and the phase angle of the sum has changed by 180 degrees.

The model prediction of the behavior detailed in Figure 3–6 for a −50 dB stimulus is typical of all stimulus amplitudes below this level. That is, there will be a sharp minimum when the gain is about 35 dB/octave. See, for example, the response for stimulus levels 60 dB below the saturation level in Figure 3–6. For much weaker stimuli, however, the emission amplitude for these cochlear amplifier gain levels drops so rapidly that this sharp minimum would not be observable in practice. For stimuli less than 50 dB below the saturation level, there is not a relative maximum observed as the cochlear amplifier gain initially decreases.

The unusual behavior at a stimulus level 40 dB below the saturation level in Figure 3–5 deserves comment. At this stimulus level, the emission at high and at low cochlear amplifier gains is mostly from the base region. However, at moderate stimulus levels (between $-60$ and $-40$ dB re: the saturation level) the peak emission exceeds the base. There would therefore be two 180-degree phase changes seen as the cochlear amplifier gain drops from 100 dB/octave to zero.

It would be possible that the complex behaviors seen at moderate stimulus levels in Figure 3–5 were limited to a few peculiar choices of stimulus levels, and not generally expected. This is not the case. An analysis of a number of different parameter choices produces very similar behavior, albeit occurring at slightly different stimulus levels. Figure 3–7 presents model results for the smaller stimulus frequency ratio $f_2/f_1 = 1.10$, in contrast to the frequency ratio $f_2/f_1 = 1.28$ in Figure 3–5. Figure 3–8, however, differs

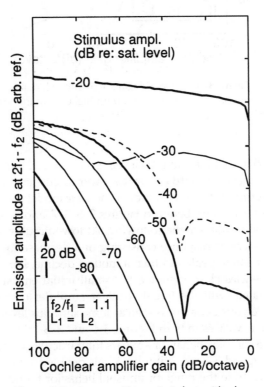

**Figure 3–7.** Same as Figure 3–5, but with closer stimulus frequencies ($f_2/f_1 = 1.1$).

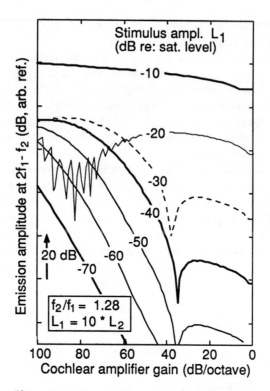

**Figure 3–8.** Same as Figure 3–5, but with different stimulus levels ($L_1$ is 20 dB higher than $L_2$).

from Figure 3–5 in that the stimulus levels are not equal, but the higher frequency stimulus level is 20 dB below the lower frequency level ($L_1 = 10L_2$). Note that all figures in this report are for the *same* model cochlea—only the stimulus parameters differ between Figures 3–5, 3–7, and 3–8.

The general results are the following: At low stimulus levels, there is always a characteristic response consisting of a decrease to a sharp notch followed by a relative peak and then a modest decline. For cases with the stimulus frequencies close together, the small initial emission amplitude increase associated with the initial cochlear amplifier decrease does not appear. However, this behavior is seen at some stimulus level for the wider stimulus frequency cases in both Figures 3–5 and 3–8.

Even more complex behavior appears for particular stimulus levels: In Figures 3–5, 3–7, and 3–8, the stimulus levels denoted −40, −30, and −20, respectively, illustrate the range of unusual behavior found. The behavior occurs because at the respective stimulus levels, the emissions from the base and peak regions are very similar. The difference is small and varies in a complex way as the cochlear amplifier gain varies.

Finally, at high stimulus levels there is typically a smooth, monotonic decrease in emission amplitude as cochlear amplifier gain decreases. The decrease is typically small over the entire range of cochlear amplifier gain.

## CONCLUSIONS

It has been shown that the complex behavior of distortion product emissions can be explained by a simple, consistent model of emission generation. The two key features of this model are (1) there is a simple saturation of the cochlear amplifier gain, which causes a broadening of the sharp peak in the response as the stimulus level is increased, and (2) the emissions which sum to a non-zero contribution can be considered to originate in two regions, a small region centered on the peak of the emission, and the larger region basal to this. The phase angles of the summed emissions from these two areas are assumed to be opposing. So, the difference between the emission amplitudes from the two areas constitutes the observed emission.

Normally, the sharp peak of the emission at low stimulus levels provides a larger contribution than the sum of the emissions from the base. At high stimulus levels, or at all levels when the cochlear amplifier gain is low, the emission from the peak region decreases, so that the emission summed from the base region dominates. The reduction in peak emission is due to the saturation posited in the first assumption. The model quite adequately explains the observed characteristics of the emission seen as the gain of the cochlear amplifier is decreased by acute furosemide intoxication. This includes the characteristic modest, monotonic decline at high stimulus levels, and the sharp minimum observed at low stimulus levels, associated with a phase angle change of 180 degrees.

At all levels and at all times, the summed emission amplitudes from each of the two regions are comparable in total intensity. Therefore, quite complex behavior can be observed at the middle stimulus levels, where the emissions from the two regions are nearly equal in intensity. As the parameters are changed slightly, one or the other of these components may dominate, leading to a number of phase changes.

The emission model adequately explains the appearance of "active" and "passive" emission components. However, the "passive" component, as has been shown here, is not entirely passive. Strictly speaking, the component previously identified as passive is only completely passive when the cochlear amplifier gain is zero. It is, however, "continuous" with the active emission found at high stimulus levels. This has been, of course, one of the factors that has led to its identification as "passive." It may be preferable to identify the two major components by their putative regions of origin, that is, as "peak" and "base" instead of "active" and "passive."

The implications of the model results for the interpretation of distortion product otoacoustic emissions are as follows. *Complex behavior observed in emissions does not necessarily imply complex behavior in the mechanics of the cochlea.* To avoid possible complications, emission measurements should be taken at a sequence of stimulus levels, that is, at the least for a complete growth function for one stimulus frequency and intensity ratio. Absolute emission levels at the lower stimulus levels give the most sensitive indication of cochlear function. The model results therefore confirm previous conclusions in this regard (e.g., Rübsamen et al., 1995).

*Changes* in emissions amplitudes at high stimulus levels also may provide an unambiguous (but less sensitive) indicator of cochlear function. The results from high stimulus levels could be potentially very useful for cases of moderate to severe cochlear amplifier dysfunction, when low stimulus level emissions are no longer measurable, *provided* the experimental paradigm allows for a difference measurement to be made, that is, a within-animal comparison. The changes in the absolute emission levels for high level stimuli are too small for this to be very useful for between group comparisons.

It is the emissions for moderate stimulus levels, within 10–20 dB of the stimulus where a "notch" is frequently observed, that cannot be used as accurate indicators of cochlear function. At these stimulus levels, quite complex behavior, with large changes in emission amplitude, can occur for very small changes in cochlear function. It does not seem appropriate to use this behavior as a possible "sensitive" assay for the occurrence of more subtle phenomena, for example, efferent effects. The reason is that the sensitivity of the complex behavior depends strongly, and unpredictably, on the precise stimulus conditions and cochlear parameters. For example, consider the emission amplitude as an indicator of cochlear amplifier gain in Figure 3–8. For stimulus levels in the range −30 to −10 dB below the saturation level, a small change in the effective stimulus level at the cochlea makes a very large change in the response. It seems less misleading to examine the changes in a complete growth function rather than at such a single stimulus point.

**Acknowledgement:** Support was provided by research grant DC 00395 from the National Institute on Deafness and Other Communication Disorders, National Institutes of Health.

# REFERENCES

Brown, A. M. (1987). Acoustic distortion from rodent ears: A comparison of responses from rats, guinea pigs and gerbils. *Hearing Research, 31,* 25–38.

Brown, A. M., & Kemp, D. T. (1985). Intermodulation distortion in the cochlea: Could basal vibration be the major cause of round window CM distortion? *Hearing Research, 19*, 191–198.

Brown, A. M., McDowell, B., & Forge, A. (1989). Acoustic distortion products can be used to monitor the effects of chronic gentamicin treatment. *Hearing Research, 42*, 143–156.

Johnstone, B. M., Gleich, B., Mavadat, N., McAlpine, D., & Kapadia, S. (1990). Some properties of the cubic distortion tone emission in the guinea pig. *Advances in Audiology, 7*, 57–62.

Kemp, D. T., & Brown, A. M. (1984). Ear canal acoustic and round window electrical correlates of $2f_1–f_2$ distortion generated in the cochlea. *Hearing Research, 13*, 39–46.

Kujawa, S. G., & Liberman, M. C. (1996). *Sound conditioning enhances cochlear responses in guinea pig.* Paper presented at the nineteenth midwinter research meeting of the Association for Research in Otolaryngology, St. Petersburg Beach, FL.

Liberman, M. C., Puria, S., & Guinan, J. J. (1996). *The ipsilaterally evoked olivocochlear reflex causes rapid adaption of the $2f_1–f_2$ DPOAE.* Paper presented at the nineteenth midwinter research meeting of the Association for Research in Otolaryngology, St. Petersburg Beach, FL.

Lonsbury-Martin, B. L., Martin, G. K., Probst, R., & Coats, A. C. (1987). Acoustic distortion products in rabbit ear canal. I. Basic features and physiological vulnerability. *Hearing Research, 28*, 173–189.

Mills, D. M. (1997). Interpretation of distortion product otoacoustic emission measurements. I. Two stimulus tones. *Journal of the Acoustical Society of America, 102*, 413–429.

Mills, D. M., Norton, S. J., & Rubel, E. W. (1993). Vulnerability and adaptation of distortion product otoacoustic emissions to endocochlear potential variation. *Journal of the Acoustical Society of America, 94*, 2108–2122.

Mills, D. M., Norton, S. J., & Rubel, E. W. (1994). Development of active and passive mechanics in the mammalian cochlea. *Auditory Neuroscience, 1*, 77–99.

Mills, D. M., & Rubel, E. W. (1994). Variation of distortion product otoacoustic emissions with furosemide injection. *Hearing Research, 77*, 183–199.

Mills, D. M., & Rubel, E. W. (1996). Development of the cochlear amplifier. *Journal of the Acoustical Society of America, 100*, 428–441.

Norton, S. J., Bargones, J. Y., & Rubel, E. W. (1991). Development of otoacoustic emissions in gerbil: Evidence for micromechanical changes underlying development of the place code. *Hearing Research, 51*, 73–92.

Nuttall, A. L., & Dolan, D. F. (1996). Steady-state sinusoidal responses of the basilar membrane in guinea pig. *Journal of the Acoustical Society of America, 99*, 1556–1565.

Probst, R., Lonsbury-Martin, B. L., & Martin, G. K. (1991). A review of otoacoustic emissions. *Journal of the Acoustical Society of America, 89*, 2027–2067.

Puel, J.-L., & Rebillard, G. (1990). Effect of contralateral sound stimulation on the distortion product $2f_1–f_2$: Evidence that the medial efferent system is involved. *Journal of the Acoustical Society of America, 87*, 1630–1635.

Rebillard, G., & Lavigne-Rebillard, M. (1992). Effect of reversible hypoxia on the compared time courses of endocochlear potential and $2f_1–f_2$ distortion products. *Hearing Research, 62*, 142–148.

Robles, L., Ruggero, M. A., & Rich, N. C. (1986). Basilar membrane mechanics at the base of the chinchilla cochlea. I. Input-output functions, tuning curves, and response phases. *Journal of the Acoustical Society of America, 80,* 1364–1374.

Rübsamen, R., Mills, D. M., & Rubel, E. W. (1995). Effects of furosemide on distortion product otoacoustic emissions and on neuronal responses in the anteroventral cochlear nucleus. *Journal of Neurophysiology, 74,* 1628–1638.

Schmiedt, R. A., & Adams, J. C. (1981). Stimulated acoustic emissions in the ear canal of the gerbil. *Hearing Research, 5,* 295–305.

Smoorenburg, G. F. (1972). Audibility region of combination tones. *Journal of the Acoustical Society of America, 52,* 603–614.

Whitehead, M. L., Lonsbury-Martin, B. L., & Martin, G. K. (1992a). Evidence for two discrete sources of $2f_1$–$f_2$ distortion-product otoacoustic emission in rabbit. I: Differential dependence on stimulus parameters. *Journal of the Acoustical Society of America, 91,* 1587–1607.

Whitehead, M. L., Lonsbury-Martin, B. L., & Martin, G. K. (1992b). Evidence for two discrete sources of $2f_1$–$f_2$ distortion product otoacoustic emission in rabbit. II: Differential physiological vulnerability. *Journal of the Acoustical Society of America, 92,* 2662–2682.

Williams, D. M., & Brown, A. M. (1995). Contralateral and ipsilateral suppression of the $2f_1$–$f_2$ distortion product in human subjects. *Journal of the Acoustical Society of America, 97,* 1130–1140.

# Otoacoustic Emissions for the Study of Auditory Function in Infants and Children

*Yvonne S. Sininger, Ph.D.*
*Carolina Abdala, Ph.D.*
Children's Auditory Research Laboratory
House Ear Institute
Los Angeles, California

It is not exaggeration to say that the discovery of otoacoustic emissions (OAEs) by David Kemp has revolutionized the study of the auditory system. The impact on the field of auditory system development and clinical assessment of hearing in infants and children has been especially dramatic. The isolated cochlear site of OAE generation has allowed the first reliable discrimination of cochlear and neural function in the developing human auditory system. The ease and reliability of OAE measurement in infants has revitalized national interest in newborn infant hearing screening. In addition, implementation of a clinical instrument for reliable recordings of OAEs has brought this technique rapidly into clinical practice, allowing for increased sophistication in differential diagnosis of complex auditory disorders in children.

## OTOACOUSTIC EMISSIONS IN INFANTS AND CHILDREN

Under ideal recording conditions, spontaneous, transient-evoked, and distortion-product otoacoustic emissions are easily recorded from infants and children with normal cochlear (and conductive) auditory function. Newborns generally have larger OAEs than adults with higher frequency spectral content than adults (Norton & Widen, 1990). This may reflect differences in the dimensions and resonance characteristics of the middle ear and ear canal of newborns. Larger emissions in neonates may also reflect the output of healthy, uncontaminated cochleae as emission strength has been shown to decline with age even after changes in ear size and resonance are complete (Norton & Widen, 1990).

The study of spontaneous otoacoustic emissions (SOAEs) in neonates provides fascinating insight into the developing ear. SOAEs are very narrow-band signals that are generated in the cochlea without auditory simulation, or spontaneously. They occur most often between about 500 and 3000 Hz and range in level from a few dB above the noise floor of measurement (–10 dB or so) to as high as 30 dB SPL. Generally, the prevalence of SOAEs is as high, or higher in neonates (Abdala, 1996; Burns, Arehart, & Campbell, 1992; Kok, Van Zanten, & Brocarr, 1993; Morlet, et al., 1995; Strickland, Burns, & Tubis, 1985) than in adults. The number and/or level of SOAEs is often greater in newborns than in adults (Burns et al., 1992; Kok et al., 1993). Perhaps most interesting are trends that show that prevalence, number of peaks, and overall level of infant SOAEs are greater in right than left ears and greater in female than male subjects (Burns et al., 1992; Kok et al., 1993; Strickland et al., 1985). These findings vary across study and occasionally interactions between gender and ear are also noted. Implications and interpretations of these trends are not yet clear. However, measurement of SOAEs has clearly elucidated some of these subtle trends in development of cochlear function.

## AUDITORY SYSTEM DEVELOPMENT

Although the principal application of otoacoustic emissions in humans has been in the hearing clinic, they are also being utilized as noninvasive probes of human cochlear physiology. OAEs are a preneural (cochlear) phenomenon; they remain intact when afferent auditory fibers are severed (Siegel & Kim, 1982), or chemically blocked (Arts, Norton, & Rubel). Further evidence of the preneural nature of this phenomenon is revealed when increasing stimulus rate, which does not cause OAE fatigue as one would expect of a neural response (Gerling & Finitzo-Hieber, 1983). Finally, in documented cases of neural pathology, OAEs are generally not affected (Bonfils & Uziel, 1988). For these reasons, OAEs can be applied to measure isolated cochlear function.

Scientists are severely limited in the techniques available for assessment of auditory function in human neonates. Prior to the discovery and description of OAEs, auditory development was evaluated primarily via assessment of auditory behaviors (Bargones, Werner, & Marean, 1995; Werner & Bargones, 1991; Werner & Marean, 1991) or by means of auditory evoked potentials, primarily the auditory brainstem response (ABR)

(Collet et al., 1987; Eggermont & Salamy, 1988; Folsom, 1985; Klein, 1986; Salamy, Mendelson, Tooley, Chaplin, 1980; Starr & Amlie, 1981). Although behavioral and evoked potential assessments provided valuable information regarding the development of hearing in the newborn period, they involve many levels of the auditory system, including the cochlea and neural structures simultaneously. Consequently, it was not possible to discern the developmental time course of peripheral (cochlear) mechanisms from more central (brainstem and auditory cortex) structures until otoacoustic emissions were available.

Many aspects of the auditory brainstem response, including amplitude, latency, interpeak latency, and waveform morphology, continue to mature well after the first year of life. We now realize that synaptic and axonal maturation have similar time courses and are reflected in ABR indices. Auditory functions, for example, tuning as measured by means of ABR, reflect these immaturities (Abdala & Folsom, 1995a, 1995b).

The most recent work on human auditory system development, summarized below, utilizes OAEs to specifically study human cochlear development. These data reveal for the first time that, in contrast to the auditory system as a whole, the auditory periphery appears to be fully mature at birth. These conclusions could not have been reached without a reliable, noninvasive assessment tool, the otoacoustic emission.

## Development of Cochlear Frequency Resolution

### Distortion Product OAE Suppression Tuning Curves

Suppression techniques have been used to describe the tuning characteristics of OAEs. Suppression is demonstrated when the cochlear response (OAE) is reduced by the introduction of a suppressor stimulus that falls within certain frequency boundaries (Harris & Glattke, 1992). In the late 1970s and early 1980s Kemp (1979) and Kemp and Chum (1980) described suppression patterns for transient-evoked otoacoustic emissions (TEOAEs) and stimulus frequency emissions to establish that the response was physiological and not simply an artifact. More recently, suppression has been used with distortion-product otoacoustic emissions (DPOAEs) to investigate cochlear frequency resolution.

DPOAE suppression occurs when a third tone is presented simultaneously with the two primary tones ($f_1$, $f_2$) and varied in level until a specified reduction in DPOAE amplitude occurs. Plotting suppressor level necessary to produce this criterion reduction (typically around 6 dB) by suppressor frequency reveals a DPOAE iso-suppression tuning curve (STC) (see Figure 4–1). Suppression tuning curves have been generated in nonhuman species (Abdala, Sininger, Ekelid, & Zeng, 1996; Brown & Kemp, 1984; Frank & Kössl, 1995; Harris & Glattke, 1992; Köppl & Manley,

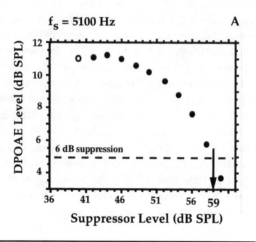

$f_s = 5100$ Hz        **A**

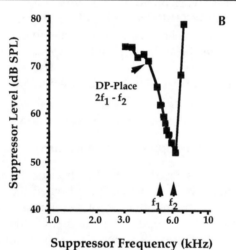

**B**

**Figure 4–1. A.** DPOAE level as a function of suppressor level. As the suppressor level is raised in 2-dB steps, DPOAE amplitude decreases. The dashed horizontal line and arrow indicate which suppressor level corresponds to 6-dB suppression in DPOAE. **B.** Once the appropriate suppressor level that causes 6=dB amplitude reduction is identified, it is plotted as a function of suppressor frequency. When this process is repeated for 10 to 15 suppressor tones of different frequency, a DPOAE iso-suppression tuning curve (STC) is generated.

1993; Martin, Lonsbury-Martin, Probst, Scheinin, & Coats, 1987), human adults (Abdula, Sininger, Ekelid, & Zeng; Harris, Probst, & Zu; Kummer, Janssen, & Arnold, 1995), Sininger, Jewett, Gardi, & Morris, 1987) and more recently, in human neonates (Abdala et al., 1996; Abdala & Sininger, 1996). Results thus far suggest that DPOAE STCs provide a measure of cochlear tuning around $f_2$, which is considered the DPOAE generation site. Measures of tuning curve width, slope, tip level, and frequency can be derived from DPOAE generation site. Measures of tuning curve width, slope, tip level, and frequency can be derived from DPOAE suppression tuning curves.

Developmental studies of DPOAE suppression generated from our laboratory (Abdala et al., 1996; Abdala & Sininger, 1996) have shown that DPOAE suppression tuning curve width, shape, and slope are adultlike in human neonates at term-birth (see Figure 4–2). These results strongly suggest that the cochlea is tuned in an adultlike manner at birth. In contrast, previous work using the ABR to evaluate tuning reported non-adult-like tuning curves until approximately 6 months of age, probably due to neur-

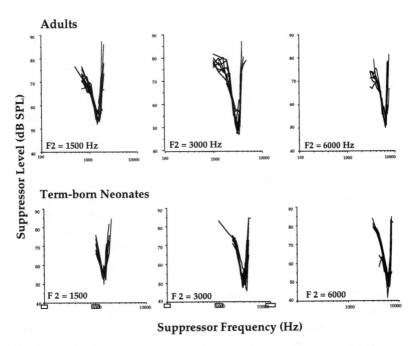

**Figure 4–2.** Twenty-eight DPOAE suppression tuning curves recorded from 15 normal-hearing adults and 29 DPOAE suppression tuning curves recorded from 26 healthy, term-born neonates at three $f_2$ frequencies: (a) 1500, (b) 3000, and (c) 6000 Hz. Tuning curve width, slope, tip level, and frequency are comparable in adult and neonatal subjects.

al, rather than cochlear, immaturity (Abdala & Folsom, 1995a; Folsom & Wynne, 1987). Ongoing work in our lab includes the generation of DPOAE STCs in premature neonates to define the developmental time course for the maturation of cochlear tuning. Although the DPOAE iso-suppression technique requires continued investigation and experimental replication, it holds promise as a noninvasive means of evaluating cochlear frequency resolution in humans.

Suppression has also been used with spontaneous and transient OAEs to probe cochlear develpment. Bargones and Burns (1988) generated SOAE suppression tuning curves in infants 2–3 weeks of age and, consistent with our results, found that infant tuning curve width and slope values fell within the adult range for all frequencies. Folsom and Burns (1994) generated transient-evoked suppression tuning curves in adults and 3-month-old infants and found comparable tuning curve shape between ages as well.

### Distortion Product OAE $f_2/f_1$ Frequency Ratio Functions

When DPOAE amplitude is plotted as a function of $f_2/f_1$ frequency ratio, a typical, bandpass-shaped function is generated that appears to reflect cochlear filtering (Abdala, 1996; Allen & Fahey, 1993; Brown & Gaskill, 1990; Brown, Gaskill, Carlyon, & Williams, 1993). This bandpass function is similar to a tuning curve in many ways; it becomes narrower with increased frequency, and broadens as stimulus level decreases. Several investigators have suggested that this function can give an indication of frequency selectivity in the human cochlea and have found a correlation between psychophysical measures of tuning and $f_2/f_1$ frequency ratio (FR) functions (Allen & Fahey, 1993; Brown et al., 1993).

Our laboratory recently conducted a study of the $f_2/f_1$ FR function in premature and term-born human neonates to determine optimal frequency ratio for DPOAE testing in infants and to investigate cochlear development (Abdala, 1996). Our findings show that the shape, width, and slope of the frequency ratio function in human adults, term neonates, and premature neonates were comparable at both low and high frequencies. This finding provides further evidence that cochlear function is mature early in human development.

DEVELOPMENT OF BASILAR MEMBRANE TRAVEL TIME. Eggermont and colleagues (Eggermont, Brown, Ponton, & Kimberley, 1996) have applied DPOAE latency and phase information to derive estimates of cochlear traveling wave time in human adults and neonates (Eggermont et al., 1996). DPOAE phase measurements reflect the time from stimulus onset to DPOAE generation around $f_2$, filter response delay at this site, and reverse transmission back toward the stapes. This measurement of travelling wave delay is related to cochlear tuning in that the width and sharpness of the auditory filter at or near $f_2$ will influence travel time. Consistent with findings of adultlike DPOAE suppression tuning curves and $f_2/f_1$ FR functions prior to term-birth in human neonates, traveling wave delay data indicate mature cochlear functioning at 35 weeks gestational age. Any age-related differences observed can be adequately explained by standing wave interference in the measurement of stimulus level at the tympanic membrane of adult subjects.

**DEVELOPMENT OF THE COCHLEAR AMPLIFIER.** In small mammals, the growth function of the DPOAE (DPOAE amplitude × stimulus level) has proven to be a valuable tool for studying the development of active processes within the cochlea termed the *cochlear amplifier* (Mills, Norton, & Rubel, 1994; Mills & Rubel, 1996; Whitehead, Lonsbury-Martin, & Martin, 1992a, 1992b). The cochlear amplifier is thought to sharpen cochlear frequency resolution and enhance auditory sensitivity primarily for low-level sounds (Davis, 1983; Neely & Kim, 1983). Outer hair cell integrity and the presence of a high endocochlear potential are critical to cochlear amplifier function (Brown, McDowell, & Forge, 1989; Norton, Bargones, Rubel, 1991; Ruggero & Rich, 1991). Precise details of cochlear amplifier function during human development remain largely unknown.

The cochlear amplifier saturates with moderate to high-level stimuli. Consequently, generation of distortion with high-level stimuli is thought to be a product of passive basilar-membrane mechanics rather than cochlear amplifier activity. Because of this, the DPOAE growth function offers a tool for differentiating between cochlear activity based in active processes and activity dominated by passive vibration of the basilar membrane. The low-level segment of the function has been shown to be vulnerable to outer-cell damage, reduction of the endocochlear potential, and anoxia in small mammals. The high-level segment represents passively dominated movement and is generally unaffected by manipulations known to affect the cochlear amplifier (see Figure 4–3) (Brown et al., 1989; Norton, Bargones, & Rubel, 1991; Whitehead et al., 1992a, 1992b).

In humans, the DPOAE growth function has not been well characterized or studied in depth. The few studies conducted thus far have shown high variability in shape and slope among human DPOAE growth functions (Lonsbury-Martin & Martin, 1990). Human functions appear to be adequately described, in most cases, by a straight line rather than the typical two-segment shape observed in small mammals (Popelka, Karzon, & Arjmand, 1995; Popelka, Osterhammel, Nielsen, & Rasmussen, 1993). However, the human DPOAE growth function has not been studied with the objective of delineating active from passive cochlear function. Ongoing work in our lab is delving into this question. We are generating DPOAE growth functions from human adults and neonates under various stimulus conditions in an effort to detect whether active and passive modalities of

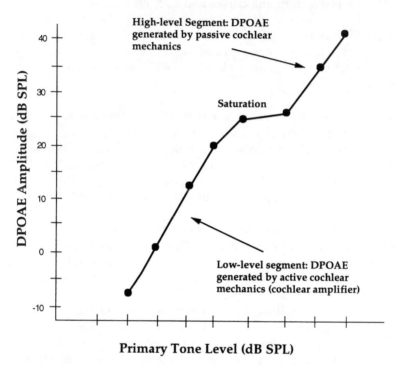

# DPOAE Growth Function

**High-level Segment: DPOAE generated by passive cochlear mechanics**

**Saturation**

**Low-level segment: DPOAE generated by active cochlear mechanics (cochlear amplifier)**

DPOAE Amplitude (dB SPL)

Primary Tone Level (dB SPL)

**Figure 4–3.** A schematic DPOAE growth function or plot of amplitude as a function of stimulus level. In small mammals, there are two segments to the mature growth function: a low-level segment that is thought to reflect distortion generated by active cochlear mechanics and a high-level segment reflecting distortion dominated by passive basilar membrane mechanics. These two segments are separated by a flattened region reflecting a transition between active and passive response modalities.

distortion generation exist in humans. If these modalities are present, the DPOAE growth function may offer a window into development of the cochlear amplifier in the human auditory system.

In conclusion, within the last decade, novel techniques of OAE generation, measurement, and application have been applied to humans and have provided access to a once forbidden portion of the human auditory system: the cochlea. These techniques must be carefully tested and validated in human subjects before we accept their application and value; however, there appears to be general agreement that otoacoustic emissions hold enormous potential for probing development, function, and dysfunction of the human cochlea.

# CLINICAL APPLICATIONS OF OAES IN INFANTS AND CHILDREN

Otoacoustic emissions achieved the status of a routine audiologic clinical procedure very soon after the phenomenon was initially described in 1978. By the mid-1990s most clinics were using OAEs routinely and billing codes were issued. The reason for the rapid acceptance of this technique must be due, in part, to the development of a machine that produced OAEs with careful controls on response accuracy and reliability. The ILO88®, followed by the ILO92® (Bray & Kemp, 1987), incorporated measurement techniques such as dual intertwined OAE measures used automatically for estimates of replicability to estimate signal strength and difference measures to estimate response noise, meters showing growth of response strength, ear canal measures of stimulus characteristics with feedback for user adjustment and monitoring of stimulus stability over recording time, automatic spectral analysis of response as well as display of time waveform for immediate detection, and many other features. These features, which we have come to expect on any OAE measurement device, led to nearly foolproof measures, an important aspect to transition of experimental techniques into clinical practice. This contribution by Kemp and colleagues must be included when we list his accomplishments and contributions to the field of audition.

## Applications of OAE to Screening for Neonatal Hearing Loss

Soon after the initial description of otoacoustic emissions (Kemp, 1978) the possibility of applying this technique to the screening of newborns for cochlear hearing loss became a reality. The studies by Johnsen, Elberling, and colleagues (Johnsen, Bagi, & Elberling, 1983; Elberling, Parbo, Johnsen, & Bagi, 1985) demonstrated that OAEs could be recorded from virtually 100% of normally hearing, cooperative, full-term neonates. These findings created a great wave of enthusiasm for using this rapid, reliable technique sensitive to mild cochlear hearing loss as a new method for screening of all neonates for cochlear dysfunction.

Published results of clinical studies utilizing TEOAEs for evaluating or screening of auditory function in newborns show wide discrepancies in experimental protocol. A summary of experimental protocols and results of these studies can be found in Table 4–1. All studies involving large numbers of infants published at the time of this writing have utilized transient stimuli to evoke an otoacoustic emission. Many of these studies have employed the nonlinear click (Kemp, Bray, Alexander, & Brown, 1986; Norton & Neely, 1987) to reduce stimulus artifact, but screening stimulus level varies somewhat and the level referent (nHL or SPL) is not consistent. Generally, clicks of 30 to 45 dB nHL or 70 to 85 dB SPL are employed in infants for mild to moderate hearing loss. There is a clear need for more consistent

**Table 4-1.** Summary of OAE studies on infants.

| Study | Stimulus | Level | Max | Environment | Hours Postpartum | Pass Criteria | Fail Result | %Pass Normal | No. of Babies/Ears |
|---|---|---|---|---|---|---|---|---|---|
| Kennedy et al. (1991) | Click | 26 & 36 dB nHL | Not given | Not given | Not given | Fsp > 2.0 and Corr. ≥ .5 | Retest -> ABR | (26 dB) 95% (36 dB) 97% | 714 ears Norm+ High risk+ NICU |
| Elberling et al. (1985) | 2 kHz Click | 70 & 50 dB (32.5 & 12.5 dB p.e. SPL) | 800 | Not given | 48–96 hrs | Amp &/or Corr > Control | N/A | 100% | 100 Norm |
| Stevens et al. (1987) | Linear and Nonlinear Clicks | 31 & 41 dB nHL | 1000 | Sound-treated chamber | Mean = 69 hrs (Normals) | Visual corr. of 2 traces aided by R | N/A | (41) 83% (31) 81% Normals: (41) 96% | 30 Norm 112 NICU |
| White et al. (1993) | Click | Not given | Not given | Quiet room Closed isolette | 24–48 hrs (Normals) | 3 dB SNR in 1–4 kHz | Retest OAE & ABR | 73% Stage One | 1546 Norm 304 NICU |
| Salomon et al. (1992) | Nonlinear Click | 69 dB SPL | 1000 2X | Quiet room | 8 hours to 8 days | Response shape, spectra, and SNR | Retest | 93% (one ear) 86% (both ears) | 209 Norm |
| Uziel & Piron (1991) | Linear and Nonlinear Clicks | 70 dB SPL (32.5 dB nHL) | 2 @ 250 | Quiet room or sound isolated chamber | 1–5 days | Not stated | ABR | 97% N 79% Risk | 55 Norm 40 NICU |

| Study | Stimulus | Intensity | Number | State | Age | Pass criteria | Confirmation | Pass rate | Subjects |
|---|---|---|---|---|---|---|---|---|---|
| Brass et al. (1994) | Nonlinear Click | 71–81 dB SPL | 520 | Not given | 3–6 weeks | SNR in 1.6–2.8 kHz QUIKSCRN | Not given | 79% (QS) 72% RI comp. pass | 82 Norm |
| Bonfils et al. (1990) | Clicks | 30 dB nHL | 2048 | Natural sleep | 21 hrs–4 days | Repeatability saturation or response at X frequency | Not given | 90% day 1 100% day 4 98% overall | 52 Norm (100 ears) |
| Hunter et al. (1994) | Clicks | 31 & 41 dB nHL | 500 | On ward with monitored sound levels | 24–95 hrs | Fsp >2 & R > .5 | ABR | 78% (both ears) 83% (one ear) | 201 risk, NICU + Norm |

standards for stimulus type and level employed when OAE methods are applied to screening of auditory function in newborns. Evaluation of the use of DPOAEs for newborn hearing screening should also be addressed.

Test environment also varies considerably across studies, as illustrated in Table 4–1, from bedside to sound-isolated chambers. Infant status (full-term newborns or intensive care unit infants) and mix also varied across studies and contributed significantly to discrepancy in results. Perhaps most inconsistent of the variables across studies, is the criteria used to distinguish those infants who have a present OAE and "pass" the screening from those who "fail." It is most common to employ the techniques employed in the ILO system designed by Kemp, Bray, Alexander, and Brown (1986) such as dual trace storage for visual and computational cross correlation or comparison of the estimated OAE level with or without comparison to estimated recording noise level (RMS level for difference waveform). Given the wide discrepancies in study design, the variability in percentage of infants who are able to "pass" a newborn screening using OAEs is not surprising (see Table 4–1).

## Middle and External Ear Influence on OAEs

Studies of infant OAEs have found that results can be contaminated in infants evaluated immediately after birth and that the percentage of babies showing a robust OAE increases dramatically during the first few days postpartum (Kok, Van Zanten, & Brocaar, 1992). It appears that naturally occurring early contamination of the external ear canal by debris such as vernix casseosa as well as the status of the aeration of the middle ear can disrupt the normal recording of OAEs especially in the first 24 hours after birth.

Data from our lab (Sininger, Cone-Wesson, & Ma, 1993) show that neonatal click-evoked ABR peak latencies rapidly diminish over the first 5 days postpartum and that the percentage of the same full-term babies with a robust OAE improves dramatically after about 30 hours (see Figure 4–4). The I–V interpeak interval does not change during this same period indicating that these rapid changes are most likely indicative of conductive mechanism changes rather than neural or cochlear function. These data and others indicate the presence of early, rapid changes in the ears of newborns that influence the percentage of infants who will display a clear OAE.

Immediately after birth the ear canal of infants is often contaminated by debris including vernix. The amount of ear canal obstruction due to this substance appears to diminish rapidly over the first 3 days (Cavanaugh, 1996) as this substance is naturally worked out of the ear. Vernix can impede the recording of OAEs in newborns by occluding the ear canal, diminishing the OAE-eliciting signal level and/or the OAE itself which is measured in the ear canal. It is also possible that the ports in the recording probe become blocked by ear canal debris. Chang, Vohr, Norton, and Lekas

## DAYS ONE THROUGH FIVE POSTPARTUM

### ABR LATENCY

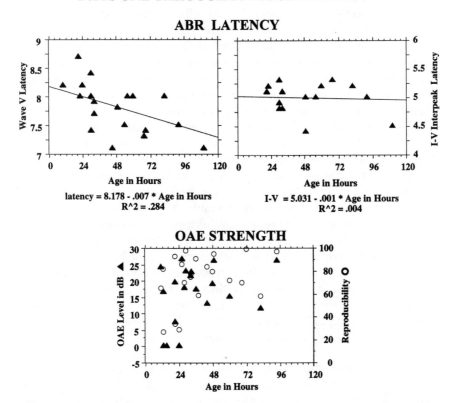

**Figure 4–4.** Otoacoustic emissions measured with 80 dB SPL nonlinear clicks using an ILO-88 and ABR measured in response to 60 dB nHL clicks in a group of full-term neonates ranging in age from 10 to 188 hours postpartum. Each data point represents the data from a single infant collected in a cross-sectional manner. Some infants were evaluated by both OAE and ABR. I–V latencies do not change substantially indicating that changes in the conductive mechanism are most likely responsible. OAE data show that, prior to 30 hours of age, some infants show poor OAE amplitude and reproducibility whereas after that time all infants demonstrated a robust response.

(1993) found that swabbing the ear canal of neonates who averaged 43 hours old dramatically improved the number of infants in whom a robust OAE could be recorded. Our own experience with newborn OAE recording has shown that, when an OAE is not seen, removal of the probe and clearing of any occluding debris often allow for a clean OAE recording.

Normal changes in the status of the middle ear over the first days postpartum are more difficult to document and less clearly understood. Northrop, Piza, and Eavey (1986) have shown evidence of residual amniotic fluid in the middle ear space of neonatal temporal bones. By studying bones obtained up to 70 days of age, they show that the amniotic cellular tissue seems to be removed over time by cellular processes.

The presence of such substance in the middle ear could be responsible for attenuation of either eliciting stimuli or of the OAE itself as it is conducted through the middle ear to be measured in the ear canal. Thornton, Kimm, Kennedy, and Cafarelli-Dees (1993) have shown that the percentage of full-term infants displaying normal tympanograms increases from just over 50% on day 1 to close to 100% by day 3 postpartum. At the same time the middle ear pressure is reduced from about 20 daPa to about 3 daPa. Abnormal reduced compliance and positive pressure would be consistent with the presence of amniotic fluid in the middle ear.

Although naturally occurring changes in the ear of normal neonates may reduce the overall pass rate of OAEs during the first few hours after birth, these obstacles are not insurmountable. Attenuation in eliciting stimuli can be overcome by increasing stimulus levels within reasonable guidelines. Also, OAEs in neonates are known to be larger in amplitude than those of adults (Norton & Widen, 1990) often reaching 30 dB or more. The amplitude of these responses will increase the likelihood that a newborn OAE will be able to be recorded through minor attenuation due to increased middle ear stiffness. Clearing of the ear canals or measurement probes and waiting 24 hours or more after birth to make recordings should also reduce the incidence of false positive results when using OAEs for infant screening.

Enthusiasm for the use of OAEs in newborn screening is reflected in the action of the National Institute of Health, whose 1993 Consensus Conference on Early Identification of Hearing Impairment in Infants and Young Children recommended establishing programs for "universal" neonatal hearing screening and even suggested a test battery that begins with otoacoustic emissions. The National Institute on Deafness and Other Communicative Disorders also funded a 5-year project to study the details of using otoacoustic emissions and auditory brainstem response for newborn auditory screening. This renewed level of interest in neonatal hearing screening can be directly attributed to the discovery of the phenomenon known as otoacoustic emissions by David Kemp.

## OAEs for Prediction of Hearing Level

The aspect of OAEs that makes them uniquely suited to infant screening is the fact that the response will disappear with more than a mild degree of cochlear hearing loss. In his initial description, Kemp (1978) reported that TEOAEs could be expected to be absent in any persons with hearing loss greater than 30 dB, and in a subsequent study (Bray & Kemp, 1987) he found that all of 79 infants and children had present TEOAEs if their hearing loss was less than 20 dB. Others have reported that the upper limit of hearing loss was less than 20 dB. Others have reported that the upper limit of hearing loss in neonates who have detectable TEOAEs is approximately 40 dB (Bonfils, 1989; Bonfils, Uziel, & Pujol, 1988). DPOAEs in response to high-level primary tones have been seen in frequency regions with hearing thresholds as high as 60 dB (Lonsbury-Martin & Martin, 1990). In the hands of those with considerable experience, a clear relationship between stimulus sensation level and OAE amplitude (input-output function) can be discerned for given subjects (Lonsbury-Martin & Martin, 1990) at least up to the SL at which the OAE disappears. However, in light of the large variability in amplitude across subjects, it is unlikely that hearing threshold could be predicted with accuracy from individual measurements of OAE. The presence of an OAE to a moderate-level stimulus is excellent for ruling out significant (mild or greater) peripheral hearing impairment but more conclusions cannot be drawn. Prediction of thresholds when hearing loss exists will have to rely on other techniques.

## OAEs for Differential Diagnosis of Auditory Disorders

There is increasing evidence that a substantial subset of infants and children with hearing loss and auditory dysfunction may have normal cochlear function with auditory nerve and brainstem dysfunction, a condition termed *Auditory Neuropathy* (Sininger, Hood, Starr, Berlin, & Picton, 1995; Starr et al., 1991; Starr, Picton, Sininger, Hood, & Berlin, 1996). It is noteworthy that prior to the time when otoacoustic emissions were available in audiology clinics for assessment of these cases, the etiology and site of lesion of this disorder were not clearly understood (Kraus, Ozdamar, Stein, & Reed, 1984; Worthington & Peters, 1980). Bilateral auditory nerve disorder leading to significant hearing loss was not accepted as a clinical entity until clear evidence of normal cochlear function (in this case outer hair cell function) was demonstrated by the presence of otoacoustic emissions in these patients.[1] The finding of other evidence of peripheral neuropathy in these patients (Starr et al., 1996) has led us to the conclusion that the auditory nerve is a more likely site of lesion for this disorder than the inner hair cell or inner hair cell-auditory nerve synapse.

The widespread use of otoacoustic emissions in the clinic has shown us that auditory neuropathy is more widespread than we would have once imagined (Berlin et al., 1993; Gravel & Stapells, 1993; Katona et al., 1993; Lutman, Mason, Sheppard, & Gibbin, 1989; McGee, Kraus, Killion, Rosenberg, & King, 1993; Welzl-Müller, Stephan, & Stadlmann, 1993) and is pre-

---

[1] In our initial description of a patient with what we termed "synchrony disorder" (Starr et al., 1991) we had evidence of normal outer hair cell function from measures of cochlear microphonics. This was confirmed with otoacoustic emissions just before publication. Measurements of cochlear microphonics are not made routinely in the clinic and often require sedation.

sent in patients of all ages including newborns (Stein et al., 1996). Differential diagnosis of this disorder, which is easily misdiagnosed as cochlear impairment, is crucial because traditional rehabilitation methods such as hearing aids are both ineffective (Sininger et al., 1995) and contraindicated by the presence of normal hair-cell function. Alternative rehabilitation strategies, typically using visual or tactile modes of stimulation, must be used with theses children until other treatments are found.

In summary, the discovery of the phenomenon known as otoacoustic emissions by David Kemp has truly revolutionized the study of audition. It has dramatically advanced study and knowledge of general cochlear processes which enhance frequency selectivity and sensitivity. Not only has this technique enhanced our understanding of normal cochlear processes, it has provided us with an objective, accurate, and simple assessment tool for studying these processes, which are fully developed in humans at the time of birth. In addition, we can study the development of cochlear processes in premature human infants to increase our understanding of the time course of such development.

In the clinic, we can credit Dr. Kemp with providing accurate, fast assessment tools for the detection of cochlear dysfunction and hearing loss in the youngest infants. It is clear that the discovery of the phenomenon of OAE as well as the implementation of hardware and software for accurate assessment of the phenomenon have revitalized interest in universal screening for hearing loss in neonates. The ultimate impact of early detection of hearing loss cannot be completely assessed but will certainly have far-reaching implications for those children for whom hearing loss is detected in the newborn period rather than later in life.

We can also look to OAEs as a quick and accurate assessment tool for children for the detection of mild hearing loss and for the differential diagnosis of cochlear and neural dysfunction. Again, the importance of this distinction cannot be fully realized at this time but we should see a dramatic change in our ability to provide early, appropriate rehabilitation for hearing loss in all children throughout the coming decade.

# REFERENCES

Abdala, C. (1996). DPOAE ($2f_1$–$f_2$) amplitude as a function of $f_2/f_1$ frequency ratio and primary tone level separation in human adults and neonates. *Journal of the Acoustical Society of America, 100*(6), 3726–3740.

Abdala, C., & Folsom, R. (1995a). The development of frequency resolution in humans as revealed by the auditory brain-stem response recorded with notched-noise masking. *Journal of the Acoustical Society of America, 98*, 921–930.

Abdala, C., & Folsom, R. C. (1995b). Frequency contribution to the click-evoked auditory brain-stem response in human adults and infants. *Journal of the Acoustical Society of America, 97*, 2394–2404.

Abdala, C., & Sininger, Y. S. (1996). The development of cochlear frequency resolution in the human auditory system. *Ear and Hearing, 17*(5), 374–385.

Abdala, C., Sininger, Y. S., Ekelid, M., & Zeng, F.-G. (1996). Distortion product otoacoustic emission suppression tuning curves in human adults and neonates. *Hearing Research, 98*, 38–53.

Allen, J. B., & Fahey, P. F. (1993). A second cochlear-frequency map that correlates distortion product and neural tuning measurements. *Journal of the Acoustical Society of America, 94*, 809–816.

Arts, H. A., Norton, S. J., & Rubel, E. W. (1990). Influence of perilymphatic tetrodotoxin and calcium concentration on hair cell function. *ARO Abstracts, 194*.

Bargones, J. Y., & Burns, E. M. (1988). Suppression tuning curves for spontaneous otoacoustic emissions in infants and adults. *Journal of the Acoustical Society of America, 83*, 1809–1816.

Bargones, J. Y., Werner, L. A., & Marean, G. C. (1995). Infant psychometric functions for detection: Mechanisms of immature sensitivity. *Journal of the Acoustical Society of America, 98*, 99–111.

Berlin, C. I., Hood, L. J., Wen, H., Cecola, R. P., Rigby, P., & Jackson, D. F. (1993). Contralateral suppression of non-linear click-evoked otoacoustic emissions. *Hearing Research, 71*, 1–11.

Bonfils, P. (1989). Spontaneous otoacoustic emissions: Clinical interest. *Laryngoscope, 99*, 752–756.

Bonfils, P., & Uziel, A. (1988). Evoked otoacoustic emissions in patients with acoustic neuromas. *American Journal of Otolaryngology, 9*, 412–417.

Bonfils, P., Dumont, A., Marie, P., Francois, M., & Narcy, P. (1990). Evoked otoacoustic emissions in newborn hearing screening. *Laryngoscope, 100*, 186-189.

Bonfils, P., Uziel, A., & Pujol, R. (1988). Screening for auditory dysfunction in infants by evoked oto-acoustic emissions. *Archives of Otolaryngology—Head and Neck Surgery, 114*, 887–890.

Brass, D., Watkins, P., & Kemp, D. T. (1994). Assessment of implementation of a narrow band, neonatal otoacoustic emission screening method. *Ear and Hearing, 15*(6), 467–475.

Bray, P., & Kemp, D. T. (1987). An advanced cochlear echo technique suitable for infant screening. *British Journal of Audiology, 21*, 191–204.

Brown, A. M., & Gaskill, S. A. (1990). Measurement of acoustic distortion reveals underlying similarities between human and rodent mechanical responses. *Journal of the Acoustical Society of America, 88*, 840–849.

Brown, A. M., Gaskill, S. A., Carlyon, R. P., & Williams, D. M. (1993). Acoustic distortion as a measure of frequency selectivity: Relation to psychophysical equivalent rectangular bandwith. *Journal of the Acoustical Society of America, 93*, 3291–3297.

Brown, A. M., & Kemp, D. T. (1984). Suppressibility of the $2f_1$-$f_2$ stimulated acoustic emissions in gerbil and man. *Hearing Research, 13*, 29–37.

Brown, A. M., McDowell, B., & Forge, A. (1989). Acoustic distortion products can be used to monitor the effects of chronic gentamicin treatment. *Hearing Research, 42*, 143–156.

Brown, A. M., Sheppard, S. L., & Russell, P. T. (1994). Acoustic distortion products (ADP) from the ears of term infants and young adults using low stimulus levels. *British Journal of Audiology, 28*, 273–280.

Burns, E. M., Arehart, K. H., & Campbell, S. L. (1992). Prevalance of spontaneous otoacoustic emissions in neonates. *Journal of the Acoustical Society of America, 91,* 1571–1575.

Cavanaugh, R. M. J. (1996). Pneumatic otoscopy in healthy full-term infants. *Pediatrics, 79,* 520–523.

Chang, K. W., Vohr, B. R., Norton, S. J., & Lekas, M. D. (1993). External and middle ear status related to evoked otoacoustic emission in neonates. *Archives of Otolaryngology—Head and Neck Surgery, 119,* 276–282.

Collet, L., Delorme, C., Chanal, J. M., Dubreuil, C., Morgon, A., & Salle, B. (1987). Effect of stimulus intensity variation on brain-stem auditory evoked potentials: Comparison between neonates and adults. *Electroencephalography and Clinical Neurophysiology, 68,* 231–233.

Dallos, P. (1973). *The auditory periphery. Anonymous.* New York: Academic Press.

Davis, H. (1983). An active process in cochlear mechanics. *Hearing Research, 9,* 79–90.

Eggermont, J. J., Brown, D. K., Ponton, C. W., & Kimberley, B. P. (1996). Comparison of DPE and ABR travelling wave delay measurements suggests frequency specific synapse maturation. *Ear and Hearing, 17*(5), 386–394.

Eggermont, J. J., & Salamy, A. (1988). Maturational time course for the ABR in preterm and full infants. *Hearing Research, 33,* 35–48.

Elberling, C., Parbo, J., Johnsen, N. J., & Bagi, P. (1985). Evoked acoustic emission: Clinical application. *Acta Oto-Rhio-Laryngologica (Stockholm), 421*(Suppl.), 77–85.

Folsom, R. C. (1985). Auditory brain stem responses from human infants: Pure-tone masking profiles for clicks and filtered clicks. *Journal of the Acoustical Society of America, 78,* 555–562.

Folsom, R. C., & Burns, E. M. (1994). Transient-evoked otoacoustic emission and auditory brainstem response suppression tuning curves in human adults and infants. *ARO Abstracts, 17,* 51.

Folsom, R. C., & Wynne, M. K. (1987). Auditory brain stem responses from human adults and infants: Wave V tuning curves. *Journal of the Acoustical Society of America, 81,* 412–417.

Frank, G., & Kössl, M. (1995). The shape of $2f_1$-$f_2$ suppression tuning curves reflects basilar membrane specializations in the mustached bat, *Pteronotus parellii. Hearing Research, 83,* 151–160.

Gerling, I. J., & Finitzo-Hieber, T. (1983). Auditory brainstem response with high stimulus rates in normal and patient populations. *Annals of Otology, Rhinology and Laryngology, 92,* 119–123.

Gravel, J. S., & Stapells, D. R. (1993). Behavioral, electrophysiologic, and otoacoustic measures from a child with auditory processing dysfunction: Case report. *Journal of the American Academy of Audiology, 4,* 412–419.

Harris, F. P., & Glattke, T. J. (1992). The use of suppression to determine the characteristics of otoacoustic emissions. *Seminars in Hearing, 13,* 67–79.

Harris, F. P., Probst, R., & Xu, L. (1992). Suppression of the $f_1$–$f_2$ otoacoustic emission in humans. *Hearing Research, 64,* 133–141.

Hunter, M. F., Kimm, L., Cafarelli-Dees, D., Kennedy, C. R., & Thornton, A. R. D. (1994). Feasibility of otoacoustic emission detection followed by ABR as a universal neonatal screening test for hearing impariment. *British Journal of Audiology, 28,* 47–51.

Johnsen, N. J., Bagi, P., & Elberling, C. (1983). Evoked acoustic emissions from the human ear. III. Findings in neonates. *Scandinavian Audiology, 12,* 17–24.

Katona, G., Buki, B., Farkas, Z., Pytel, J., Simon-Nagy, E., & Hirschberg, J. (1993). Transitory evoked otoacoustic emission (TEOAE) in a child with profound hearing loss. *International Journal of Pediatric Otorhinolaryngology, 26,* 263–267.

Kemp, D. T. (1978). Stimulated acoustic emissions from within the human auditory system. *Journal of the Acoustical Society of America, 64,* 1386–1391.

Kemp, D. T. (1979). Evidence of mechanical nonlinearity and frequency selective wave amplification in the cochlea. *Archives of Oto-Rhino-Laryngology, 224,* 37–45.

Kemp, D. T., Bray, P., Alexander, L., & Brown, A. M. (1986). Acoustic emission cochleography—Practical aspects. *Scandinavian Audiology, 25*(Suppl.), 71–95.

Kemp, D. T., & Chum, R. (1980). Properties of the generator of stimulated acoustic emissions. *Hearing Research, 2,* 213–232.

Kennedy, C. R., Kimm, D., Cafarelli-Dees, D., Evans, P. I. P., Hunter, M., Lenton, S., & Thornton, R. D. (1991). Otoacoustic emissions and auditory brainstem responses in the newborn. *Archives of Disease in Childhood, 66*(10, Spec No), 1124–1129.

Klein, A. J. (1986). Masking effects on ABR waves I and V in infants and adults. *Journal of the Acoustical Society of America, 79,* 755–759.

Kok, M. R., Van Zanten, G. A., & Brocaar, M. P. (1992). Growth of evoked otoacoustic emissions during the first days postpartum. *Audiology, 31,* 140–149.

Kok, M. R., Van Zanten, G. A., & Brocaar, M.P. (1993). Aspects of spontaneous otoacoustic emissions in healthy newborns. *Hearing Research, 69,* 115–123.

Köppl, C., & Manley, G. A. (1993). Distortion-product otoacoustic emissions in the bobtail lizard. II Suppression tuning characteristics. *Journal of the Acoustical Society of America, 93,* 2834–2843.

Kraus, N., Ozdamar, O., Stein, L., & Reed, N. (1984). Absent auditory brain stem response: Peripheral hearing loss or brain stem dysfunction? *Laryngoscope, 94,* 400–406.

Kummer, P., Janssen, T., & Arnold, W. (1995). Suppression tuning characteristics of the $2f_1$-$f_2$ distortion-product otoacoustic emission in humans. *Journal of the Acoustical Society of America, 98,* 197–210.

Lonsbury-Martin, B. L., & Martin, G. K. (1990). The clinical utility of distortion-product otoacoustic emissions. *Ear and Hearing, 11,* 144–154.

Lutman, M. E., Mason, S. M., Sheppard, S., & Gibbin, K. P. (1989). Differential diagnostic potential of otoacoustic emissions: A case study. *Audiology, 28,* 205–210.

Martin, G. K., Lonsbury-Martin, B. L., Probst, R., Scheinin, S., & Coats, A. C. (1987). Acoustic distortion products in rabbit ear canal. II Sites of origin revealed by suppression contours and pure-tone exposures. *Hearing Research, 28,* 191–208.

McGee, T., Kraus, N., Killion, M., Rosenberg, R., & King, C. (1993). Improving the reliability of the auditory middle latency response by monitoring EEG delta activity. *Ear and Hearing, 14,* 76–84.

Mills, D. M., Norton, S. J., & Rubel, E. W. (1994). Development of active and passive mechanics in the mammalian cochlea. *Auditory Neuroscience, 1,* 77–99.

Mills, D. M., & Rubel, E. W. (1996). Development of the cochlear amplifier. *Journal of the Acoustical Society of America, 100,* 428–441.

Morlet, T., Lapillonne, A., Ferber, C., Duclaux, R., Sam, L., Putet, G., Salle, B., & Collet, L. (1995). Spontaneous otoacoustic emissions in preterm neonates: Prevalance and gender effects. *Hearing Research, 90,* 44–54.

Neely, S. T., & Kim, D. O. (1983). An active cochlear model showing sharp tining and high sensitivity. *Hearing Research, 9,* 123–130.

Northrop, C., Piza, J., & Eavey, R. D. (1986). Histological observations of amniotic fluid cellular content in the ear of neonates and infants. *International Journal of Pediatric Otorhinolaryngology, 11*, 113–127.

Norton, S. J., Bargones, J. Y., & Rubel, E. W. (1991). Development of otoacoustic emissions in gerbil: Evidence of micromechanical changes underlying development of the place code. *Hearing Research, 51*, 73–92.

Norton, S. J., & Neely, S. T. (1987). Tone-burst-evoked otoacoustic emissions from normal-hearing subjects. *Journal of the Acoustical Society of America, 81*(6), 1860–1872.

Norton, S. J., & Stover, L. J. (1994). Otoacoustic emissions: An emerging clinical tool. In J. Katz (Ed.), *Handbook of clinical audiology.* (4th ed., pp. 448–462). Baltimore: Williams & Wilkins.

Norton, S. J., & Widen, J. E. (1990). Evoked otoacoustic emissions in normal-hearing infants and children: Emerging data and issues. *Ear and Hearing, 11*, 121

Popelka, G. R., Karzon, R. K., & Arjmand, E. M. (1995). Growth of the $2f_1$-$f_2$ distortion product otoacoustic emission for low-level stimuli in human neonates. *Ear and Hearing, 16*, 159–165.

Popelka, G. R., Osterhammel, P. A., Nielsen, L. H., & Rasmussen, A. N. (1993). Growth of distortion product otoacoustic emissions with primary-tone level in humans. *Hearing Research, 88*, 12–22.

Ruggero, M. A., & Rich, N. C. (1991). Furosemide alters organ of Corti mechanics: Evidence for feedback of outer hair cells upon the basilar membrane. *Journal of Neuroscience, 11*, 1057–1067.

Salamy, A., Mendelson, T., Tooley, W. H., & Chaplin, E. R. (1980). Differential development of brainstem potentials in healthy and high-risk infants. *Science, 210*, 553–554.

Salomon, G., Anthonisen, B. J., & Thomsen, P. P. (1992). Otoacoustic hearing screening in newborns: Optimization. In F. H. Bess & J. Hall (Eds.), *Screening children for auditory function* (pp. 191–206). Nashville, TN: Bill Wilkerson Center Press.

Siegel, J. H., Kim, D. O. (1982). Vulnerability to acoustic trauma and other alterations as seen in neural responses and ear-canal sound pressure. In D. Hamernik, D. Henderson, & R. Salvi (Eds.), *New perspectives on noise-induced hearing loss* (pp. 137–151). New York: Raven Press.

Sininger, Y. S., Cone-Wesson, B., & Ma, E. (1993). Auditory status of the newborn during the first days postpartum. *Abstracts of the Association for Research in Otolaryngology, 16*, 5.

Sininger, Y. S., Hood, L. J., Starr, A., Berlin, C. I., & Picton, T. W. (1995). Hearing loss due to auditory neuropathy. *Audiology Today, 7*, 10-13.

Starr, A., & Amlie, R. (1981). The evaluation of newborn brainstem and cochlear functions by auditory brainstem potentials. In R. Korobkin & C. Guilleminault (Eds.), *Progress in perinatal neurology* (pp. 65–84). Baltimore: Williams & Wilkins.

Starr, A., McPherson, D., Patterson, J., Don, M., Luxford, W. M., Shannon, R., Sininger, Y. S., Tonokawa, L. T., & Waring, M. (1991). Absence of both auditory evoked potentials and auditory percepts dependent on timing cues. *Brain, 114*, 1157–1180.

Starr, A., Picton, T. W., Sininger, Y. S., Hood, L. J., & Berlin, C. I. (1996). Auditory neuropathy. *Brain, 119*, 741–753.

Stein, L., Tremblay, K., Pasternak, J., Banerjee, S., Lindemann, K., & Kraus, N. (1996). Brainstem abnormalities in neonates with normal otoacoustic emissions. *Seminars in Hearing, 17*, 197–213.

Stevens, J., Webb, H., Smith, M., Buffin, J., & Ruddy, H. (1987). A comparison of otoacoustic emissions and brain stem electric response audiometry in the normal newborn and babies admitted to a special care baby unit. *Clinical Physics and Physiological Measurement, 8*, 95–104.

Strickland, E. A., Burns, E. M., & Tubis, A. (1985). Incidence of spontaneous otoacoustic emissions in children and infants. *Journal of the Acoustical Society of America, 78*, 931–935.

Thornton, A. R., Kimm, L., Kennedy, C. R., & Cafarelli-Dees, D. (1993). External- and middle-ear factors affecting evoked otoacoustic emissions in neonates. *British Journal of Audiology, 27*, 319–327.

Uziel, A., & Piron, J.-P. (1991). Evoked otoacoustic emissions from normal newborns and babies admitted to an intensive care baby unit. *Acta Oto-Rhino-Laryngologica (Stockholm), 482*(Suppl.), 85–91.

Welzl-Müller, K., Stephan, K., & Stadlmann, A. (1993). Click-evoked otoacoustic emission in a child with unilateral deafness. *European Archives of Otorhinolaryngology, 250*, 366–368.

Werner, L. A., & Bargones, J. Y. (1991). Sources of auditory masking in infants: Distraction effects. *Perception & Psychophysics, 50*, 405–412.

Werner, L. A., & Marean, G. C. (1991). Methods for estimating infant thresholds. *Journal of the Acoustical Society of America, 90*, 1867–1875.

White, K. R., Vohr, B. R., & Behrens, T. R. (1993). Universal newborn hearing screening using transient evoked otoacoustic emissions: Results of the Rhode Island hearing assessment project. *Seminars in Hearing, 14*(1), 18–29.

Whitehead, M. L., Lonsbury-Martin, B. L., & Martin, G. K. (1992a). Evidence for two discrete sources of $2f_1$–$f_2$ distortion-product otoacoustic emission in rabbit: I. Differential dependence on stimulus parameters. *Journal of the Acoustical Society of America, 91*, 1587–1607.

Whitehead, M. L., Lonsbury-Martin, B .L., & Martin, G. K. (1992). Evidence for two discrete sources of $2f_1$–$2f_2$ distortion-product otoacoustic emission in rabbit. II: Differential physiological vulnerability. *Journal of the Acoustical Society of America, 92*, 2662–2682.

Worthington, D. W., & Peters, J .F. (1980). Quantifiable hearing and no ABR: Paradox or error? *Ear and Hearing, 1*, 281–285.

# 5

# The Application of Distortion Product Otoacoustic Emissions to Identify Carriers of Recessive Hereditary Deafness

*Jer-Min Huang, M.D., Ph.D.*
*Charles I. Berlin, Ph.D.*
*Bronya J. B. Keats, Ph.D.*
*Shu-Tze Lin, M.P.H.*
*Matthew Money, M.D.*
Kresge Hearing Research Laboratory of the South
Molecular and Human Genetics Center
Louisiana State University Medical Center
New Orleans, Louisiana

About 1 of 4,000 newborns shows hereditary sensorineural deafness. Four million babies are born each year in the United States. Therefore, about 1000 people each year are born with hereditary deafness. Since roughly 60% of hereditary deafness is transmitted in an autosomal recessive mode, there are about 600 new cases of recessive deafness annually in the U.S.

It has been estimated that about 12% of the population carries a recessive deafness gene of some kind. Individuals who have one copy of the recessive deaf gene and no hearing loss are called carriers. If both parents are carriers of the same deafness gene, their children will have a one in four chance of inheriting two identical copies of the deafness gene and showing the trait. Aside from such mathematical estimates, we still cannot offer parents reliable clinical information on how likely it is that they will have one or more deaf children despite the significant progress in locating and identifying human and nonhuman deafness genes. The purpose of this chapter is to report the results of animal studies done toward developing a recording technique to identify carriers of recessive hereditary hearing impairment (Huang, Money, Berlin, & Keats, 1995, 1996; Huang, Money, Lim, & Berlin, 1997).

## HEARING LOSS DIPS IN CARRIERS

Since the 1960s, many clinicians have attempted unsucessfully to apply auditory testing to identify the carriers of recessive hereditary hearing impairment. Unproductive procedures have included pure-tone, Bekesy, and Audioscan audiometry, as well as SISI, routine ABRs, tone decay, and speech audiometry (for review, see Anderson & Wedenberg, 1968; Cohen et al., 1996; Cremers, Marres, & van Rijn, 1991; Ehret, 1976; Eldridge, Berlin, Money, & McKusick, 1968; Jaber et al., 1992; Kloepfer, Laguaite, & McLaurin, 1966; Konigsmark, 1971; Konigsmark, Hollander, & Berlin, 1968; Liu & Xu, 1994; Madell & Sculerati, 1991; Marres & Cremers, 1989; Mengele, Konigsmark, Berlin, & McKusick, 1967; Nance & McConnell, 1973; Oeken & Konig, 1993; Ruben & Rozycki, 1971; Taylor, Hine, Brasier, Chiveralls, & Morris, 1975). Although no test has been proven sufficiently effective, the results of Bekesy and Audioscan audiograms often show deep hearing loss notches in a specific frequency range in many carriers (Cohen et al., 1996; Marres & Cremers, 1989; Meredith et al., 1992). Therefore, the auditory function of carriers may reveal minor defects that are difficult to detect by pure-tone audiometry.

## OTOACOUSTIC EMISSIONS AND AUDITORY GENETICS

The discovery of otoacoustic emissions (OAEs) (Kemp, 1978) opened a new window for us to study the relationship between genetics and auditory function. The distortion product otoacoustic emission (DPOAE), a type of OAE, can be recorded in many species. The ear canal DPOAE test has provided an objective, noninvasive, and frequency-specific measure for the sensory function of the cochlea (Kemp, Ryan, & Bray, 1993; Kim, Paparello, Jung, Smurzynski, & Sun, 1996; Klattke & Kujawa, 1991; Lonsbury-Martin, McCoy, Whitehead, & Martin, 1993; Martin, Probst, & Lonsbury-Martin, 1990; Ohlms, Lonsbury-Martin, & Martin, 1990; Probst, Lonsbury-Martin, & Martin, 1991). Recently, this testing has been applied to the study of hereditary hearing loss (Lina-Granade, Collet, & Morgon, 1995) and auditory genetics (Bilger, Matthies, Hammel, & Demorest, 1990; McFadden & Loehlin, 1995).

# DISTORTION PRODUCT OTOACOUSTIC EMISSIONS (DPOAES)

The DPOAEs are generated primarily by the outer hair cells in the organ of Corti. The DPOAEs evoked by two primary tones separating appropriately are composed of multiple tones of different frequencies. The $2f_1-f_2$ DPOAE is the most robust tone measured in both human and many non-human species. Technically, the DPOAEs can be recorded as DPOAE audiograms or DPOAE input-output (I-O) functions. The DPOAE audiogram evoked by designated intensities may provide important information about cochlear function over a broad frequency range. The measure of DPOAE I-O function can further provide information about the cochlear dynamic function of a specific frequency range. The recording techniques used to develop a DPOAE test battery in our work include DPOAE audiogram and I-O function.

## DPOAE IN HEARING SCREENING

As the first step in developing a test battery to identify carriers of recessive hereditary hearing impairment, we used moderate stimulus intensity of $L_1/L_2 = 60/50$ dB SPL to record DPOAE audiograms of sound-responsive and deaf mice.

We had obtained DPOAE audiograms from 50 mice: 24 carriers of recessive hereditary deafness mice [ct(+/$dn$)] were sound-responsive with the presence of the Preyer reflex and 26 *deafness* ($dn/dn$) mice were deaf because they inherited a pair of recessive *deafness* ($dn$) genes. As expected, all of the sound-responsive mice had DPOAEs, while all of the deaf mice did not. Figure 5–1 shows the mean DPOAE audiogram of 24 sound-responsive mice. These hearing mice have well-defined DPOAE with $f_2$ frequencies between 4 and 16 kHz. Beginning at 4 kHz, the DPOAE increases rapidly to 15 dB at about 8 kHz, and then progressively increases to 30 dB at about 14 kHz. Therefore, the DPOAE amplitude as a function of $f_2$ frequency suggests that the cochleas of the normal hearing mice are more sensitive to frequencies above 4 kHz than to those below 4 kHz (Ehret, 1976; Henry, 1979; Mikaelian & Ruben, 1964).

## DPOAE PATTERNS IN GENOTYPING

Our next step was to test whether DPOAE audiogram patterns differ between hearing mouse strains. We had obtained DPOAE audiograms from three sound-responsive mouse strains: ct(+/+), CBA/J, and MOLF. The ad-

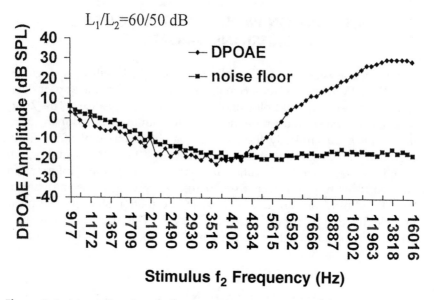

**Figure 5–1.** Mean distortion product otoacoustic emission (DPOAE) audiogram of 24 sound-responsive mice.

vantage of using these three strains is that the MOLF and CBA/J mice are different for about 90% of their respective genomes, whereas the CBA/J and ct(+/+) strains are identical for much of their genomes. Therefore, if genetic factors play a role in DPOAE patterns, then the DPOAE audiogram comparison should reflect the degree of genetic similarity among mouse strains.

Figure 5–2 displays the mean DPOAE audiograms of ct(+/+), CBA/J, and MOLF groups. As expected, the DPOAE audiogram of the ct(+/+) group is very similar to that of the CBA/J group. However, the MOLF group has smaller DPOAE amplitudes than both ct(+/+) and CBA/J groups, supporting the hypothesis that the DPOAE audiogram might permit auditory phenotyping between strains. However, when the genetic backgrounds are very close between two strains, the DPOAE audiogram evoked by the parameters used here will be less sensitive for these purposes. Therefore, we have embarked on a systematic study to refine our technique for identifying carriers and noncarriers in the same mouse strain.

## DPOAE IN IDENTIFICATION OF THE CARRIER

From our earliest work, we learned that using stimulus parameter of $L_1/L_2$ = 65 dB has its limitation in identifying carriers. As the I-O curve is characterized by two components: an active component of low inputs below 60

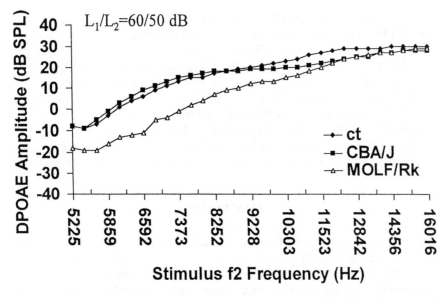

**Figure 5–2.** Mean distortion product otoacoustic emission (DPOAE) audiograms of three sound-responsive mouse strains: ct(++), CBA/J, and MOLF.

dB and a passive component of high inputs above 60 dB, the intensity level of $L_1/L_2 = 60/50$ dB we had used in previous studies is about right on the breaking point of the I-O curve and therefore is less than optimal for phenotyping carriers whose status affects the outer hair cells. Apparently, we needed a complete parametric study to extract the optimal combinations of $L_1/L_2$ intensity ratios and $f_2/f_1$ frequency ratios to allow us to best characterize the auditory systems of carriers versus noncarriers.

Therefore, we recorded DPOAE audiograms and I-O functions systematically from noncarrrier [homozygous ct(+/+)] and carrier [heterozygous ct(+/$dn$)] adult mice. The carrier and noncarrier were derived from the ct inbred strain. We have maintained this strain for more than 20 generations in our institute, thus the genomes of the carriers and noncarriers are essentially identical except that the carriers have a recessive $dn$ gene.

For the DPOAE audiogram, we used seven $L_1/L_2$ intensity levels (70/70, 60/60, 50/50, 70/60, 60/50, 60/70, and 50/60) in combination with three $f_2/f_1$ ratios (1.3, 1.2, and 1.1). For the DPOAE input-output study, all the I-O functions were recorded with a fixed $f_2$ frequency. Seven $f_2$ frequencies, ranging from 8789 Hz to 14,746 Hz, were studied (8789, 9619, 10,400, 10,986, 12,011, 13,988, 13,525, and 14,746 Hz). Each $f_2$ frequency had six stimulus conditions with different $f_2/f_1$ ratio (1.3, 1.2, or 1.1) and different relationship of $L_1$ and $L_2$ ($L_1$–$L_2$ = 0, 10, or –10 dB SPL). The input intensities were given from high to low in 1-dB steps.

As a result of this work we observed that, when the $f_2/f_1$ ratio is 1.3, the DPOAE amplitudes of carriers are larger than those of the noncarriers. This distinction is especially salient at low intensities (Figures 5–3 and 5–4).

To further confirm that the auditory trait as revealed by DPOAE is related primarily to cochlear function, we also have repeated a study reported by Kirsch, Money, and Webster (1993) showing that carriers and noncarriers have similar thresholds for the auditory brainstem response wave I evoked by clicks and tone-bursts of 1, 2, 4, 8, 16, and 32 kHz. The ABR analysis of wave I threshold and wave I latency of 50- and 70-dB stimulus-intensities showed no difference between the carriers and noncarriers.

## SUMMARY

Overall, from our studies , it can be concluded that: (a) DPOAE is useful for genetic phenotyping, (b) genetic factors play a role in DPOAE patterns, (c) the DPOAE and other auditory responses may reflect the traits of carriers of genes for recessive hearing impairment, and (d) using DPOAE testing to identify a carrier requires a 1.3 ratio and very low intensity levels.

**Acknowledgments:** This work was supported by NIH NIDCD P01-DC00379, T-32-DC0007, Kam's Fund for Hearing Research, the Louisiana Lions Eye Foundation, and Deafness Research Foundation.

## REFERENCES

Anderson, H., & Wedenberg, E. (1968). Audiometric identification of normal hearing carriers of genes for deafness. *Acta Otolaryngologica, 65,* 535–554.

Anderson, H., & Wedenberg, E. (1976). Identification of normal hearing carriers of genes for deafness. *Acta Otolaryngologica, 83,* 245–248.

Bilger, R. C., Matthies, M. L., Hammel, D. R, & Demorest, M. E. (1990). Genetic implications of gender differences in the prevalence of spontaneous otoacoustic emissions. *Journal of Speech and Hearing Research, 33,* 418–432.

Bock, K. R., & Steel, K. P. (1983). Inner ear pathology in the deafness mutant mouse. *Acta Otolaryngologica, 96,* 39–47.

Cohen, M., Francis, M., Luxon, L. M., Bellman, S., Coffey, R., & Pembery, M. (1996). Dips on Bekesy or audioscan fail to identify carriers of autosomal recessive non-syndromic hearing loss. *Acta Otolaryngologica (Stockholm), 116,* 521–567.

Cremers, C. W. R. J., Marres, H. A. M., & van Rijn, P. M. (1991). Nonsyndromal profound genetic deafness in childhood. *New York Academy of Sciences, 630,* 191–196.

Deol, M. S., & Kocher, W. (1958). A new gene for deafness in the mouse. *Heredity, 12,* 463–466.

Ehret, G. (1976). Development of absolute auditory thresholds in the house mouse (mus musculus). *Journal of the American Auditory Society, 1,* 179–184.

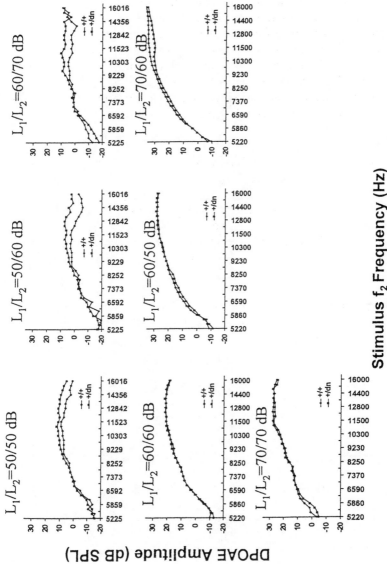

**Figure 5–3.** DPOAE differences between carriers and noncarriers are largest at *low* intensities.

133

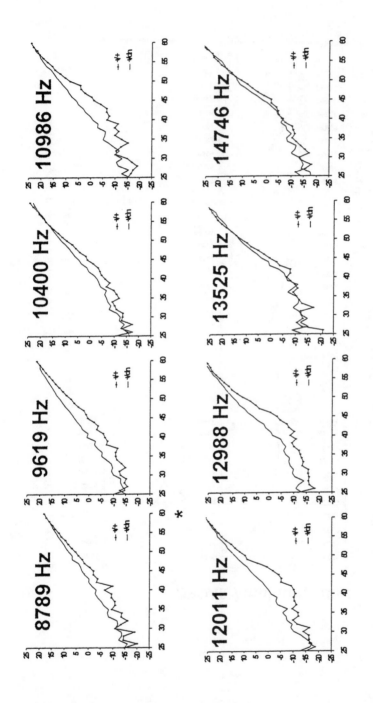

**Figure 5–3.** I-O differences between carriers and noncarriers are largest at *low* intensities.

Eldridge, R., Berlin, C. I., & Money, J. W., & McKusick, V.A. (1968). Cochlear deafness, myopia, and intellectual impairment in an Amish family. *Journal of the American Medical Association, 88,* 75–80.

Glattke, T. J., & Kujawa, S. G. (1991). Otoacoustic emissions. *American Journal of Audiology, 1,* 29–40.

Henry, K. R. (1979). Auditory nerve and brain stem volume-conducted potentials evoked by pure-tone pips in the CBA/J laboratory mouse. *Audiology, 18,* 93–108.

Horner, K. C., Lenoir, M., & Bock. G. R. (1985). Distortion product otoacoustic emissions in hearing-impaired mutant mice. *Journal of the Acoustical Society of America, 78,* 1603–1611.

Huang, J. M., Money, M. K., Berlin, C. I., & Keats, B. J. B. (1995). Auditory phenotyping of heterozygous sound-responsive (+/*dn*) and deafness (*dn/dn*) mice. *Hearing Research, 88,* 61–64.

Huang, J. M., Money, M. K, Berlin, C. I., & Keats, B. J. B. (1996). Phenotypic patterns of distortion product otoacoustic emission in inbred and F1 hybrid hearing mouse strains. *Hearing Research, 98,* 18–21.

Huang, J. M., Berlin, C. I., Lin, S. T., & Keats, B. J. B. (In press). DPOAE's at low intensities and 1.3 ratio distinguish normal hearing (+/+) from +/dn mice. *Hearing Research.*

Jaber, L., Shohat, M., Bu, X., Fischel-Ghodsian, N., Yang, H. Y., Wang, S. J., & Rotter, J. I.. (1992). Sensorineural deafness inherited as a tissue specific mitochondria disorder. *Journal of Medical Genetics, 29,* 86–90.

Keats, B. J. B, Nouri, N., Huang, J. M., Money, M. K., Webster, D. B., & Berlin, C. I. (1995). The deafness locus (*dn*) maps to mouse Chromosome 19. *Mammalian Genome, 6,* 8–10.

Kemp, D. T. (1978). Stimulated acoustic emissions from within the human auditory system. *Journal of the Acoustical Society of America, 64,* 1386–1391.

Kemp, D. T., Ryan, S., & Bray, P. (1993). A guide to the effective use of otoacoustic emissions. *Ear and Hearing, 11,* 93–105.

Kim, D. O., Paparello, J., Jung, M. D., Smurzynski, J., & Sun, X. (1996). Distortion product otoacoustic emission test of sensorineural hearing loss performance regarding sensitivity, specificity and receiver operating characterisitics. *Acta Otolaryngologica (Stockholm), 116,* 3–11.

Kirsch, J. P., Money, M. K., & Webster, D. B. (1993). Mice heterozygous for the deafness gene have normal auditory thresholds. *Hearing Research, 67,* 51–54.

Kloepfer, H. W., Laguaite, J. K., & McLaurin, J. W. (1966). The hereditary syndrome of congenital deafness and retinitis pigmentosa (Usher's syndrome). *Laryngoscope, 76,* 850–862.

Konigsmark B., W., Hollander, M. B., & Berlin, C. I. (1968). Familial neural hearing loss and atopic dermatitis. *Journal of the American Medical Association, 204,* 953–957.

Konigsmark, B.W. (1971). Hereditary congenital severe deafness syndromes. *Annals of Otology, Rhinolology, and Laryngology, 80,* 269–288.

Lina-Granade, G., Collet, L., & Morgon, A. (1995). Physiopathological investigations in a family with a history of unilateral hereditary deafness. *Acta Otolaryngologica. 115,* 196–201.

Liu, X., & Xu, L. (1994). Nonsyndromic hearing loss: An analysis of audiograms. *Annals of Otology, Rhinology, and Laryngology, 103,* 428–433.

Lonsbury-Martin, B. L., McCoy, M. C., Whitehead, M. L., & Martin, G. K. (1993). Clinical testing of distortion-product otoacoustic emissions. *Ear and Hearing, 1,* 11–22.

Madell, J. R., & Sculerati, N. (1991). Noncongenital hereditary hearing loss in children. *Archives of Otolaryngology—Head and Neck Surgey, 117,* 332–335.

Martin, G. K, Probst, R., & Lonsbury-Martin, B. L. (1990). Otoacoustic emissions in human ears: Normative findings. *Ear and Hearing, 11,* 106–120.

McFadden, D., & Loehlin, J. C. (1995). On the heritability of spontaneous otoacoustic emissions: A twin study. *Hearing Research, 85,* 181–198.

Marres, H. A. M., & Cremers, C. W. R. J. (1989). Autosomal recessive nonsyndromal profound childhood deafness in a large pedigree. *Archives of Otolaryngology—Head and Neck Surgery, 115,* 591–595.

Mengel, M. C., Konigsmark, B. W., Berlin, C. I., & McKusick, V. A. (1967). Recessive early-onset neural deafness. *Acta Otolaryngologica, 64,* 313–326.

Meredith, R., Stephens, D., Sirimanna, T., Meyer-Bisch, C., & Reardon, W. (1992). Audiometric detection of carriers of Usher's syndrome type II. *Journal of Audiology and Medicine, 1,* 11–19.

Mikaelian, D. O., & Ruben, R. J. (1964). Development of hearing in the CBA/J mouse. *Acta Otolaryngologica, 59,* 451–461.

Nance, W. E., & McConnell, F. E. (1973). Status and prospects of research in hereditary deafness. In H. Harris & K. Hirschorn (Eds.), *Advances in human genetics* (Vol. 4, pp. 175–250). New York: Plenum Press.

Oeken, J., & Konig, E. (1993). Forms of monosymptomatic hereditary sensorineural hearing loss and deafness in the Leipzig area. *HNO, 41,* 301–310.

Ohlms, L. A., Lonsbury-Martin, B. L., & Martin, G. K. (1990). The clinical application of acoustic distortion products. *Otolaryngology—Head and Neck Surgery, 103,* 52–59.

Probst, R., Lonsbury-Martin, B. L., & Martin, G. K. (1991). A review of otoacoustic emissions. *Journal of the Acoustical Society of America, 89,* 2027–2067.

Pujol, R., Schnerson, A., Lenoir, M., & Deol, M. S. (1983). Early degeneration of sensory and ganglion cells in the inner ear of mice with uncomplicated genetic deafness (dn): Preliminary observations. *Hearing Research, 122,* 57–63.

Ruben, R. J., & Rozycki, D. L. (1971). Clinical aspects of genetic deafness. *Annals of Otology, Rhinology, and Laryngology, 80,* 255–263.

Steel, K. P., & Bock, G. R. (1980). The nature of inherited degeneration in deafness mouse. *Nature, 288,* 159–161.

Taylor, I. G., Hine, W. D, Brasier, V. J., Chiveralls, K., & Morris, T. (1975). A study of the causes of hearing loss in a population with special reference to genetic factors. *Journal of Laryngology and Otology, 89,* 899–914.

Webster, D. B. (1992). Degeneration followed by partial regeneration of the organ of Corti in deafness (*dn/dn*) mice. *Experimental Neurology, 115,* 27–31.

# 6

# The Role of Otoacoustic Emissions in Identifying Carriers of Hereditary Hearing Loss

*Linda J. Hood, Ph.D.*
Kresge Hearing Research Laboratory of the South
Department of Otorhinolaryngology and Biocommunication
Louisiana State University Medical Center
New Orleans, Louisana

Hearing impairment can be the consequence of a broad range of environmental, medical, and hereditary factors. Understanding the factors underlying hereditary hearing loss is based on locating the genes that cause hearing loss and defining the specific mechanisms and functions of those genes. Much genetic research worldwide is directed toward finding the chromosome locations of genes that cause hearing loss and determining their molecular properties and functions. Study of both individuals with hereditary hearing losses and family members who are carriers of genes for those hearing losses may also contribute to the understanding of the functional characteristics of genes. Several studies reviewed in this chapter suggest that, in addition to the hearing losses exhibited by affected individuals, carriers of genes for hearing loss may have subtle auditory anomalies even though their auditory function is clinically normal.

From a clinical standpoint, understanding the characteristics of hereditary hearing loss and the impact of genetic factors on hearing may improve management strategies for individuals with hereditary hearing loss and their families. Furthermore, understanding the ways in which genes control development and function of the auditory system may, in the future, allow the influence of genetic factors that produce hearing loss to be counteracted.

This chapter discusses work that has been directed toward the evaluation of individuals who are carriers of genes for hearing loss. One group of these individuals who can be readily identified is the normal-hearing parents and siblings of individuals who have hereditary hearing loss. Auditory evaluation of parents and other nonaffected family members can be accomplished with a number of behavioral and physiological measures. Because the majority of hereditary hearing losses are sensory in nature and involve abnormal development of the receptor cells (hair cells) of the inner ear, otoacoustic emissions may be a particularly sensitive and valuable measure.

## INHERITANCE OF HEARING LOSS

Abnormal genes are a major cause of severe hearing impairment, particularly hearing impairment that occurs at a young age. Approximately 65% of cases of hereditary hearing impairment are autosomal recessive and 33% are autosomal dominant, whereas X-linked and mitochondrial defects account for 2% of cases. Recessive hearing loss is the focus of much research because it is the most common type of hereditary hearing loss and because it is less easy to predict than hearing loss resulting from a dominant inheritance pattern.

To display a recessive trait, a person must acquire one abnormal gene for the trait from each parent. Parents are heterozygous for the trait as they each carry one abnormal and one normal gene. Thus, recessively inherited defects appear among the offspring of phenotypically normal parents who both are carriers of a single recessive gene for the trait. When both parents are carriers, the chances of a child receiving two copies of the gene and therefore showing the phenotype are one in four, or 25%. Their chance of having carrier children is 50%, and of having a child with no gene for the defect is 25%. In cases of recessive hearing loss that is nonsyndromic, the nature of the disorder is obvious only in families with multiple (two or more) occurrences of the disorder. In families with only one child with the disorder it is difficult, if not impossible, to distinguish them from sporadic nongenetic cases of deafness (Nance & Sweeney, 1975).

Hereditary hearing loss comprises about one half of all cases of severe hearing loss in children and the recessive subgroup is the largest (Anderson & Wedenberg, 1968). Hereditary hearing losses range from moderate to profound (Nance & Sweeney, 1975) and autosomal recessive and sex-linked losses tend to be more severe than autosomal dominant hearing losses (Liu & Xu, 1994). The shape of the audiogram does not appear useful in differentiating between groups, although most autosomal recessive patients show residual low-frequency hearing or sharply sloping audiograms. Hereditary hearing loss can also be progressive and, in humans, onset and progression may occur in infancy and childhood. Although early degeneration at the cellular level of the organ of Corti has been observed in mice shortly after birth and prior to onset of hearing, comparable data are not available in humans.

## STUDIES OF CARRIERS OF HEREDITARY HEARING LOSS IN HUMANS

Anderson and Wedenberg (1968) and Parving (1978) summarized the literature of the 1960s and 1970s on obligate carriers of recessive hearing loss. Anderson and Wedenberg (1968, 1976) reported a "dip" in the audiometric contour using continuous frequency Bekesy audiometry, and a higher incidence of elevated stapedial reflexes in heterozygous carriers than in controls that could not be ascribed to an exogenous cause such as noise exposure or medical history. Both authors reported that Bekesy audiometry was a "poor method," but better than none, for identifying heterozygous carriers; the reported "dips" in the continuous frequency audiogram collected via Bekesy audiometry would be overlooked in standard octave band audiometry.

Another set of studies examined obligate carriers of three separate types of recessive deafness (Eldridge, Berlin, Money, & McKusick, 1968; Konigsmark, Hollander, & Berlin, 1968; Mengel, Konigsmark, Berlin, & McKusick 1967). These studies investigated Bekesy audiometry, short increment sensitivity index (SISI), tone decay tests, electrocochleography, middle ear muscle reflexes, and reflex decay. In these studies and a companion study (Konigsmark, Mengel, & Haskins, 1970), no audiologic measures were consistently abnormal in obligate carriers of genes for deafness. This failure to find reliable audiologic abnormalities in normal hearing obligate carriers has been reiterated regularly in the literature (e.g., Jaber, Shohat, Bu, Fischel-Ghodsian, Yang, Wang, & Rotter, 1992; Konigsmark, 1971, 1972a, 1972b; Liu & Xu, 1994; Madell & Sculerati, 1991; Nance & McConnell, 1973; Oeken & Konig, 1993; Ruben & Rozycki, 1971; Taylor, Hine, Brasier, Chiveralls, & Morris, 1975).

Techniques using microstructural audiometric analysis have shown some, though inconsistent, promise. Meredith, Stephens, Sirimanna, Meyer-Bisch, and Reardon (1992) used a computerized sweep frequency technique to test carriers of recessive hearing loss associated with Usher syndrome type II and found audiometric notches in the 500- to 3000-Hz frequency range. Marres and Cremers (1989) found unexplainable slight losses, attributable neither to noise damage nor presbycusis, in 3 of 12 probable carriers of autosomal recessive deafness. Stephens, Meredith, Sirimanna, France, Almqvist, and Haugen (1995) reported notches in 55% of parents of children with nonsyndromal recessive hearing loss compared to notches in 14.2% of control subjects. Stephens et al. (1995) suggested that the fact that notches did not occur invariably may be taken as a reflection of the heterogeneity of the subjects included in the sample.

Addressing genetic factors related to progressive hearing loss is also important as the genetic nature of late onset hearing loss can often be overlooked (e.g., Paparella & Schachern, 1991; Suga, Naunton, Maitland, & Hedberg, 1976; Taylor et al., 1975). Sjostrom and Anniko (1990) suggested that heterozygous jerker mice with normal hearing ultimately show widely individual variations in auditory brainstem responses (ABRs) as they age. Others suggested that a genetic predisposition must be present for such factors as rubella (Anderson, Barr, & Wedenberg, 1970) and aminoglycosides (Hu et al., 1991) to induce hearing loss, cochlear anomalies (e.g., Phelps, King, & Michaels, 1994) and concomitant visual defects. Cagini, Menduno, Ricci, Molini, and Pennachi (1995) have recently reported that 60% of normal hearing patients with retinitis pigmentosa and 24% of their relatives have abnormal otoacoustic emissions. They noted that during embryologic development there is a transitory axoneme in the outer hair cells of the organ of Corti that assists in the development and organization of the stereocilia and is present in a few mature hair cells including the photoreceptors. They cited this evidence, along with the correlation of the high incidence of emission abnormalities in the patients and their relatives, to support the notion that retinitis pigmentosa may be traceable to a structural anomaly of the ciliated cells.

## POSSIBLE GENETIC FACTORS
## RELATED TO OTOACOUSTIC EMISSIONS

Otoacoustic emissions are widely used in humans and animals to study cochlear function and the effects of the efferent system on cochlear processes. The origin of otoacoustic emissions is ascribed to processes associated with the mechanical motion of the outer hair cells, thought to be modulated through the efferent auditory pathways via the olivocochlear system (Kemp, 1978; Kemp & Chum, 1980).

Genetic factors may have a role in otoacoustic emissions. In studies of twins, McFadden and Loehlin (1995) found that the number of spontaneous otoacoustic emissions (SOAEs) was more highly correlated in monozygotic twins than in same-sex dizygotic twins. Their analyses suggested that about three quarters of the individual variation in the expression of SOAEs is attributable to genes. In addition, Bilger, Matthies, Hammel, and Demorest (1990) suggest that the tendency for females to display more SOAEs than males may be related to a dominant X-linked trait. In studies of mice, Huang, Money, Berlin, and Keats (1995) found differences in distortion product emission patterns in different strains of mice that were crossed with mice with the deafness (*dn*) gene. Keats et al. (1995) localized the *dn/dn* gene for deafness to chromosome 19 in the mouse, and Huang, Money, Berlin, and Keats (1996) showed that the pattern of high frequency DPOAEs can help distinguish between normal hearing carriers versus noncarriers of the *dn* gene. These genetic implications in humans and in mice as well as our observations in humans suggest that otoacoustic emissions are more sensitive to genetic differences than methods previously studied.

Genetic bases for specific aspects of cochlear function are further linked in that outer hair cells have a large myosin component and myosin genes are implicated in certain types of deafness (Weil et al., 1995). Because outer hair cell turgor and perhaps contractility may be related to myosin, subclinical aberrations in cochlear function might be linked to the presence of such genes.

# THE EFFERENT SYSTEM AND
# SUPPRESSION OF OTOACOUSTIC EMISSIONS

Anatomical and physiological evidence supports the interdependent function of the two ears mediated through the efferent neural pathways. The olivocochlear bundle (OCB), first described by Rasmussen (1946), has been outlined into medial (MOC) and lateral (LOC) components (Warr & Guinan, 1978; Warr, Guinan, & White, 1986). Data suggest that medial efferent fibers primarily innervate the outer hair cells, and that the hair cells contract in the presence of OCB stimulation or contralateral sound (e.g., Guinan & Gifford, 1988a, 1988b; Mountain, 1980; Siegel & Kim, 1982; Warr et al., 1986).

The observation that OAEs are altered by presentation of stimuli to the same, opposite, or both ears has made possible study of interactions between the ears. Decreases in amplitude of OAEs with contralateral stimuli suggest that suppression results from activation of the efferent pathways that affect the cochlear processes responsible for the generation of OAEs. A number of studies have described suppression of SOAEs and TEOAEs in humans by contralateral acoustic stimuli (e.g., Berlin et al., 1993; Collet et al., 1990; Grose, 1983; Hood, Berlin, Hurley, Cecola, & Bell, 1996; Hood, Berlin, Hurley, & Wen, 1996; Mott, Norton, Neely, & Warr, 1989; Rabinowitz & Widen, 1984; Ryan, Kemp, & Hinchcliffe, 1991; Schloth & Zwicker, 1983; Veuillet, Collet, & Duclaux, 1991). Binaural noise suppresses emissions in humans much more effectively than ipsilateral noise, which in turn suppresses emissions more than contralateral noise (Berlin, Hood, Hurley, Wen, & Kemp, 1995), which is consistent with a similar finding in cat efferent studies in which binaural stimulation exceeded the effects of contralateral or ipsilateral stimulation (Liberman, Puria, & Guinan, 1996). OAE suppression also has proven useful in separating patients with auditory neuropathies from normal subjects (Berlin, Hood, Cecola, Jackson, & Szabo, 1993; Williams, Brookes, & Prasher, 1994) and provides another sensitive tool with which to probe subtle cochlear processes in patients with otherwise normal audiograms or normal emissions. Efferent suppression characteristics have also been associated with thresholds for detection in noise (Micheyl, Morlet, Giraud, Collet, & Morgon, 1995) and loudness adaptation in musicians (Micheyl, Carbonnel, & Collet, 1995).

## STUDIES OF OAES AND HEREDITARY RECESSIVE HEARING LOSS IN THE ACADIAN POPULATION

We have investigated otoacoustic emissions and efferent suppression of emissions in heterozygous carriers of genes for recessive hearing loss and homozygous controls. Our studies of carriers of recessive hearing loss focus on two populations: families with Acadian Usher syndrome type I and Acadian families with nonsyndromic recessive hearing loss.

The locus for Usher type I in the Acadian population in Louisiana was mapped to the short arm of Chromosome 11 (Smith et al., 1992) and the location of this gene was refined by analysis of further markers in the region (Keats, Nouri, Pelias, Deininger, & Litt, 1994). Thus, carriers of the Acadian Usher gene who are members of a family with an affected individual can be identified (Keats et al., 1994). Acadian nonsyndromic recessive hearing loss families are parents and members of families with at least two natural children with apparent endogenous deafness. Because of their Acadian origin and close community structure, these families are genetically more homogeneous than the population at large.

We have observed that parents who are obligate carriers of the Acadian Usher syndrome type I gene show decreased distortion product otoacoustic emission (DPOAE) amplitude in the mid-frequency range when compared with a group of age- and gender-matched control subjects. An example of DPOAEs from a matched control subject and DPOAEs from a parent of a child with Usher syndrome is shown in Figures 6–1A and 6–1B, respectively. Although this has been a consistent observation in the Acadian Usher parents, emissions in parents of at least two children with nonsyndromic recessive hearing loss have been less consistent in that some of these parents show decreased mid-frequency amplitude in DPOAEs whereas other parents do not. This is not unexpected as the parents of children with nonsyndromic recessive hearing loss may comprise a more heterogeneous population.

In normal subjects below the age of 60 years, we have consistently observed an enhancement of suppression with binaural suppressor noise compared to either ipsilaterally or contralaterally presented noise. In our hereditary hearing loss studies, we have observed efferent suppression

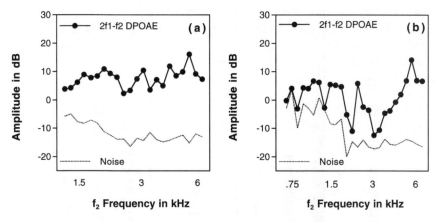

**Figure 6–1.** An example of $2f_1$–$f_2$ DPOAEs from (a) a normal control subject and (b) a normal-hearing parent of a child with Usher syndrome. Stimuli were 65 and 55 dB SPL for $f_1$ and $f_2$, respectively. The parent subject shows decreases in DPOAE amplitude, particularly in the mid-frequency range.

patterns in which binaural noise often does not enhance suppression of transient emissions to the degree observed in control subjects. The leftmost panel of Figure 6–2 shows the normal configuration of suppression where suppression with a binaural suppressor noise is the greatest, followed by suppression with an ipsilateral noise and the least suppression with a contralaterally presented suppressor. In contrast, the usual suppression pattern has not been observed in a number of the Usher and nonsyndromic recessive hearing loss parents for either one or both ears (examples in the center and right panels of Figure 6–2). In addition, across a number of carrier subjects, there appears to be less binaural enhancement than observed in normal matched control subjects.

In summary, these findings suggest that otoacoustic emissions may provide promising noninvasive methods for evaluating carriers of recessive genes for deafness. These observations in humans are consistent with findings in inbred mouse strains described in Chapter 5.

## SUMMARY

The most common forms of hereditary hearing impairment involve abnormal development of the receptor cells (hair cells) in the inner ear and follow a recessive inheritance pattern. Understanding auditory function in carriers of deafness and whether or not they display subtle differences in auditory ability may assist in understanding of the nature of genetic hearing loss and in managing individuals who carry genes for deafness but do

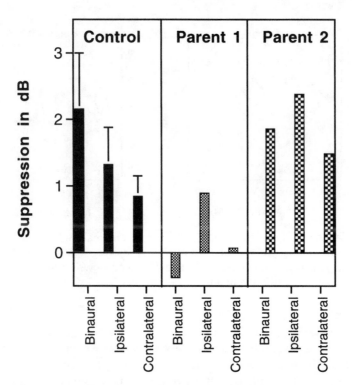

**Figure 6–2.** Efferent suppression of TEOAEs for binaural, ipsi-lateral, and contralateral noise. The leftmost panel shows the mean and one standard deviation of suppression for a group of control subjects. The center and right panels show two parents with normal hearing who are carriers of genes for recessive hearing loss. The pattern of suppression observed in control subjects is not observed in either of the parent subjects.

not exhibit the trait. The results of auditory and genetic research to characterize human genes, characterize their molecular mechanisms, and understand their function should facilitate new diagnostic and management approaches to genetic disorders.

**Acknowledgments:** This work was supported by NIH NIDCD P01-000379, Kam's Fund for Hearing Research and the Louisiana Lions Eye Foundation. Participation of Charles I. Berlin, Ph.D., Jill Bordelon, M.C.D., Leah Goforth, M.S., Annette Hurley, M.S., Bronya Keats, Ph.D., Mary Pelias, Ph.D., and Peter Rigby, M.D., in the research at Louisiana State University Medical Center on auditory aspects of hereditary hearing loss is acknowledged.

# REFERENCES

Anderson, H., Barr, B., & Wedenberg, E. (1970). Genetic disposition—A prerequisite for maternal rubella deafness. *Archives of Otolaryngology, 91*, 141–147.

Anderson, H., & Wedenberg, E. (1968). Audiometric identification of normal hearing carriers of genes for deafness. *Acta Otolaryngologica, 65*, 535–554.

Anderson, H., & Wedenberg, E. (1976). Identification of normal hearing carriers of genes for deafness. *Acta Otolaryngologica, 83*, 245–248.

Berlin, C. I., Hood, L. J., Cecola, R. P., Jackson, D. F., & Szabo, P. (1993). Does type I afferent neuron dysfunction reveal itself through lack of efferent suppression? *Hearing Research, 65*, 40–50.

Berlin, C. I., Hood, L. J., Hurley, A. E., Wen, H., & Kemp, D. T. (1995). Binaural noise suppresses linear click-evoked otoacoustic emissions more than ipsilateral or contralateral noise. *Hearing Research, 87*, 96–103.

Berlin, C. I., Hood, L. J., Wen, H., Szabo, P., Cecola, R. P., Rigby, P., & Jackson, D. F. (1993). Contralateral suppression of non-linear click-evoked otoacoustic emissions. *Hearing Research, 71*, 1–11.

Bilger, R. C., Matthies, M. L., Hammel, D. R., & Demorest, M. E. (1990). Genetic implications of gender differences in the prevalence of spontaneous otoacoustic emissions. *Journal of Speech and Hearing Research, 33*, 418–432.

Cagini, C., Menduno, P., Ricci, G., Molini, E., & Pennachi, A. (1995). Study of functionality of cochlear outer hair cells in patients with retinitis pigmentosa. *Survey of Opthalmology, 39*(Suppl. 1), S25–32.

Collet, L., Kemp, D. T., Veuillet, E., Duclaux, R., Moulin, A., & Morgon, A. (1990). Effect of contralateral auditory stimuli on active cochlear micro-mechanical properties in human subjects. *Hearing Research, 43*, 251–262.

Eldridge, R., Berlin, C. I., Money, J. W., & McKusick, V. A. (1968). Cochlear deafness, myopia, and intellectual impairment in an Amish family. *Archives of Otolaryngology—Head and Neck Surgery, 88*, 75–80.

Grose, J. H. (1983). The effect of contralateral suppression on spontaneous acoustic emissions. *Journal of the Acoustical Society of America, 74*, S38.

Guinan, J. J., & Gifford, M. L. (1988a). Mechanical and electrical coupling of efferent effects from outer hair cells to inner hair cells. *ARO Abstracts, 11*, 174.

Guinan, J. J., & Gifford, M. L. (1988b). Effects of electrical stimulation of efferent olivocochlear neurons on cat auditory-nerve fibers. III. Tuning curves and thresholds at CF. *Hearing Research, 37*, 29–46.

Hood, L. J., Berlin, C. I., Hurley, A., Cecola, R. P., & Bell, B. (1996). Contralateral suppression of transient-evoked otoacoustic emissions in humans: Intensity effects. *Hearing Research, 101*, 113–118.

Hood, L. J., Berlin, C. I., Hurley, A. E., & Wen, H. (1996). Suppression of otoacoustic emissions in normal hearing individuals. In C. I. Berlin (Ed.), *Hair cells and hearing aids* (pp. 57–72). San Diego: Singular Publishing Group.

Hu, D. N., Qui, W. Q., Wu, B. T., Fang, L. Z., Zhou, F., Gu, Y. P., Zhang, Q. H., Yan, J. H., Ding, Y. Q., & Wong, H. (1991). Genetic aspects of antibiotic induced deafness: Mitochondrial inheritance. *Journal of Medical Genetics, 28*, 79–83.

Huang, J.-M., Money, M. K., Berlin, C. I., & Keats, B. J. B. (1995). Genotype at the *dn* locus and heterosis revealed by distortion product otoacoustic emission patterns. *ARO Abstracts, 18*, 355.

Huang, J.-M., Money, M. K., Berlin, C. I., & Keats, B. J. B. (1996). Phenotypic patterns of distortion product emissions in inbred and $F_1$ hybrid hearing mouse strains. *Hearing Research, 98,* 18–21.

Jaber, L., Shohat, M., Bu, X., Fischel-Ghodsian, N., Yang, H. Y., Wang, S. J., & Rotter, J.I. (1992). Sensorineural deafness inherited as a tissue specific mitochondrial disorder. *Journal of Medical Genetics, 29,* 86–90.

Keats, B. J. B., Nouri, N., Huang, J.-M., Money, M., Webster, D. B., & Berlin, C. I. (1995). The deafness locus (*dn*) maps to mouse Chromosome 19. *Mammalian Genome, 6,* 8–10.

Keats, B. J. B., Nouri, N., Pelias, M. Z., Deininger, P. L., & Litt, M. (1994). Tightly linked flanking microsatellite markers for the Usher syndrome type I locus on the short arm of chromosome 11. *American Journal of Human Genetics, 54,* 681–686.

Kemp, D. T. (1978). Stimulated acoustic emissions from within the human auditory system. *Journal of the Acoustical Society of America, 64,* 1386–1391.

Kemp, D. T., & Chum, R. (1980). Properties of the generator of stimulated acoustic emissions. *Hearing Research, 2,* 213–232.

Konigsmark, B. W. (1971). Hereditary congenital severe deafness syndromes. *Annals of Otology, Rhinology and Laryngology, 80,* 269–288.

Konigsmark, B. W. (1972a). Genetic hearing loss with no associated abnormalities: A review. *Journal of Speech and Hearing Disorders, 37,* 89–99.

Konigsmark, B. W. (1972b). Hereditary childhood hearing loss and integumentary system disease. *Journal of Pediatrics, 80,* 909–919.

Konigsmark, B. W., Hollander, M. B., & Berlin, C. I. (1968). Familial neural hearing loss and atopic dermatitis. *Journal of the American Medical Association, 204,* 953–957.

Konigsmark, B. W., Mengel, M. C., & Haskins, H. (1970). Familial congenital moderate neural hearing loss. *Journal of Laryngology and Otology, 84,* 495–505.

Liberman, M. C., Puria, S., & Guinan, J. J. (1996). The ipsilaterally evoked olivocochlear reflex causes rapid adaptation of the $2f_1$–$f_2$ distortion product otoacoustic emission. *Journal of the Acoustical Society of America, 99,* 3572–3584.

Liu, X., & Xu, L. (1994). Nonsyndromic hearing loss: An analysis of audiograms. *Annals of Otology, Rhinology and Laryngology 103,* 428–433.

Madell, J. R., & Sculerati, N. (1991). Noncongenital hereditary hearing loss in children. *Archives of Otolaryngology—Head and Neck Surgery, 117,* 332–335.

Marres, H. A. M., & Cremers, C. W. R. J. (1989). Autosomal recessive nonsyndromal profound childhood deafness in a large pedigree. *Archives of Otolaryngology—Head and Neck Surgery, 115,* 591–595.

McFadden, D., & Loehlin, J. C. (1995). On the heritability of spontaneous otoacoustic emissions: A twins study. *Hearing Research, 85,* 181–198.

Mengel, M. C., Konigsmark, B. W., Berlin, C. I., & McKusick, V. A. (1967). Recessive early-onset neural deafness. *Acta Otolaryngologica, 64,* 313–326.

Meredith, R., Stephens, D., Sirimanna, T., Meyer-Bisch, C., & Reardon, W. (1992). Audiometric detection of carriers of Usher's syndrome type II. *Journal of Audiological Medicine, 1,* 11–19.

Micheyl, C., Carbonnel, O., & Collet, L. (1995). Medial olivocochlear system and loudness adaptation: Differences between musicians and non-musicians. *Brain and Cognition 29,* 127–136.

Micheyl, C., Morlet, T., Giraud, A. L., Collet, L., & Morgon, A. (1995). Contralateral suppression of evoked otoacoustic emissions and detection of a multi-tone complex in noise. *Acta Otolaryngologica, 115*, 178–182.

Mott, J. B., Norton, S. J., Neely, S. T., & Warr, W. B. (1989). Changes in spontaneous otoacoustic emissions produced by acoustic stimulation of the contralateral ear. *Hearing Research, 38*, 229–242.

Mountain, D. C. (1980). Changes in endolymphatic potential and crossed olivocochlear bundle stimulation alter cochlear mechanics. *Science, 210*, 71–72.

Nance, W. E., & McConnell, F. E. (1973). Status and prospects of research in hereditary deafness. In H. Harris & K. Hirschorn (Eds.), *Advances in human genetics* (Vol. 4, pp. 175–250). New York: Plenum Press.

Nance, W. E., & Sweeney, A. (1975). Genetic factors in deafness of early life. *Otolaryngologic Clinics of North America, 8*, 19–48.

Oeken, J., & Konig, E. (1993). Forms of monosymptomatic hereditary sensorineural hearing loss and deafness in the Leipzig area. *Head and Neck Otolaryngology, 41*, 301–310.

Paparella, M. M., & Schachern, P. A. (1991). Sensorineural hearing loss in children—Genetic. In M. M. Paparella, D. A. Shumrick, J. L. Gluckman, & W. L. Meyerhoff (Eds.), *Otolaryngology. Volume II. Otology and neurotology* (pp. 1579–1599). Philadelphia: W.B. Saunders.

Parving, A. (1978). Reliability of Bekesy threshold tracing in identification of carriers of genes for an X-linked disease with deafness. *Acta Otolaryngologica, 85*, 40–44.

Phelps, P. D., King, A., & Michaels, L. (1994). Cochlea dysplasia and meningitis. *American Journal of Otology, 15*, 551–557.

Rabinowitz, W. M., & Widen, G. P. (1984). Interaction of spontaneous otoacoustic emissions and external sounds. *Journal of the Acoustical Society of America, 76*, 1713–1720.

Rasmussen, G. L. (1946). The olivary peduncle and other fiber projections of the superior olivary complex. *Journal of Comparative Neurology, 84*, 141–220.

Ruben, R. J., & Rozycki, D. L. (1971). Clinical aspects of genetic deafness. *Annals of Otology, Rhinology and Laryngology, 80*, 255–63.

Ryan, S., Kemp, D. T., & Hinchcliffe, R. (1991). The influence of contralateral acoustic stimulation on click-evoked otoacoustic emissions in humans. *British Journal of Audiology 25*, 391–397.

Schloth, E., & Zwicker, E. (1983). Mechanical and acoustic influences on spontaneous otoacoustic emission. *Hearing Research, 11*, 285–293.

Siegel, J. H., & Kim, D. O. (1982). Efferent neural control of cochlear mechanics? Olivocochlear bundle stimulation affects cochlear biomechanical nonlinearity. *Hearing Research, 6*, 171–182.

Sjostrom, B., & Anniko, M. (1990). Variability in genetically induced age-related impairment of auditory brainstem response thresholds. *Acta Otolaryngologica, 109*, 353–360.

Smith, R. J. H., Lee, E. C., Kimberling, W. J., Daiger, S. P., Pelias, M. Z., Keats, B. J. B., Jay, M., Bird, A., Reardon, W., Guest, M., Ayyagari, R., & Hejtmancik, J.F. (1992). Localization of two genes for Usher syndrome type I to chromosome 11. *Genomics, 14*, 995–1002.

Stephens, D., Meredith, R., Sirimanna, T., France, L., Almqvist, C., & Haugen, H. (1995). Application of the Audioscan in the detection of carriers of genetic hearing loss. *Audiology, 34*, 91–97.

Suga, F., Naunton, R. F., Maitland, S. K., & Hedberg, K. E. (1976). Hereditary progressive sensorineural deafness. *Journal of Laryngology and Otology, 90,* 667–685.

Taylor, I. G., Hine, W. D., Brasier, V. J., Chiveralls, K., & Morris, T. (1975). A study of the causes of hearing loss in a population with special reference to genetic factors. *Journal of Laryngology and Otology, 89,* 899–914.

Veuillet, E., Collet, L., & Duclaux, R. (1991). Effect of contralateral acoustic stimulation on active cochlear micromechanical properties in human subjects: Dependence on stimulus variables. *Journal of Neurophysiology, 65,* 724–735.

Warr, W. B., & Guinan, J. J. (1978). Efferent innervation of the organ of Corti: Two different systems. *Brain Research, 173,* 152–155.

Warr, W. B., Guinan, J. J., & White, J. S. (1986). Organization of the efferent fibers: The lateral and medial olivocochlear systems. In R. A. Altschuler, R. P. Bobbin, & D. W. Hoffman (Eds.), *Neurobiology of hearing: The cochlea.* New York: Raven Press.

Weil, D., Blanchard, S., Kaplan, J., Guilford, P., Gibson, F., Walsh, J., Mburu, P., Varela, A., Levilliers, J., Weston, M.D., Kelley, P. M., Kimberling, W. J., Wagenaar, M., Levi-Acobas, F., Larget-Piet, D., Munnich, A., Steel, K. P., Brown, S. D. M., & Petit, C. (1995). Defective myosin VIIA gene responsible for Usher syndrome type 1B. *Nature, 374,* 60–61.

Williams, E. A., Brookes, G. B., & Prasher, D. K. (1994). Effects of olivocochlear bundle section on otoacoustic emissions in humans: Efferent effects in comparison with control subjects. *Acta Otolaryngologica, 114,* 121–129.

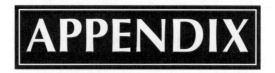

# Mathematics of Distortion Product Otoacoustic Emission Generation: A Tutorial

*Kevin H. Knuth, Ph.D.*

Dynamic Brain Imaging Laboratory
Department of Neuroscience
Albert Einstein College of Medicine
Bronx, New York

This appendix is designed to be a tutorial dealing with the mathematics of distortion products. Distortion products are typically encountered in audiology through the study of otoacoustic emissions. However, recently it has been found that auditory evoked steady-state responses can also produce distortion products (Lins & Picton, 1995). In general, distortion products can be observed in any nonlinear system that is forced to oscillate.

In this tutorial I address the following questions:

- How are distortion products produced?
- How are distortion products related to nonlinearities?
- How can distortion products be generated by transducers and microphones when they do not have hair cells?
- What do "Quadratic" and "Cubic" mean and how are these terms related to $f_2-f_1$ and $2f_1-f_2$ distortion products?
- Are there any other kinds of distortion products?

The mathematical description of distortion products will only require some basic algebra and trigonometry. The best way to approach this tutorial is to set aside a half hour and follow along using a pencil and paper. My intention is to aid you in making connections between the mathematical and physical concepts.

## LINEAR RESPONSES

Many systems oscillate: masses on springs (or rubber bands), branches in the wind, your vocal cords, guitar strings, waves on the surface of a lake, and the basilar membrane in the inner ear. Each of these systems has frequencies at which they prefer to oscillate. These frequencies are called the natural frequencies or resonance frequencies of the system. If we take any one of these systems and try to force it to oscillate at a given frequency, perhaps by shaking it, it may oscillate at a large amplitude or a small amplitude. This response amplitude depends on the relationship between the driving frequency (the frequency of our shaking) and the resonance or natural frequency of the system.

If the system is linear and we drive it with a sine wave of a given frequency, we find that it will oscillate at that frequency. Mathematically we can write the response of the system as:

$$R(t) = A(f) \ B \ Sin(2\pi ft + \varphi(f)), \tag{1}$$

where R(t) is the response or position of the system as a function of time, t is the elapsed time, f is the frequency of the stimulation or the driving frequency, A(f) is a function describing how well the system responds to the driving frequency, $\varphi(f)$ is a function describing how the phase of the response depends on the driving frequency, and B is the amplitude of the stimulation. In the equation above, we have ignored the terms describing how the response grows as it is stimulated. Instead, we will focus on the steady-state response or the long-term behavior of the system.

The idea is simple. The response of the system is essentially a sine wave at the same frequency as the driving frequency, but it is phase-shifted by an amount described by $\varphi(f)$. Its amplitude depends on the amplitude of the stimulation, B, but it also depends on how well the system responds to that frequency, A(f). If the system does not respond well at that frequency then A(f) may be quite small and the response amplitude will be quite a bit smaller than the amplitude of stimulation, B. However, if we drive it close to the resonance frequency, then A(f) may be large and the response may become larger than the stimulation amplitude. This is essentially what happens when you push someone on a swing, as long as you push at the right frequency. The function A(f) can also be visualized in terms of the basilar membrane in the cochlea. Different parts of the basilar membrane oscillate best at different frequencies and we can describe the response characteristics of each point on the basilar membrane with a function A(f).

To improve the readability of the equations we will change the notation a bit. Instead of repeatedly writing $2\pi f$, we will introduce what is called the angular frequency, $\omega$, where $\omega = 2\pi f$. This way we can write the sine function, $Sin(2\pi ft)$, above as $Sin(\omega t)$. Also we will write the frequency response as $A(\omega)$ instead of $A(f)$. Note that the functions, $A(\omega)$ and $A(f)$, are not quite the same function (actually $A(\omega) = A(2\pi f)$), but we will call both functions A just to keep the notation simple. From now on we will ignore the phase by assuming that $\varphi(f)$ is zero. With these changes, equation (1) simplifies to

$$R(t) = A(\omega) \, B \, Sin(\omega t). \tag{2}$$

The point that I want to make in this section is that the system above is linear. By linear I mean that if one doubles the amplitude of the stimulation, the magnitude of the response amplitude doubles, if one triples the stimulation amplitude, the magnitude of the response amplitude triples, and so on. In addition, if one stimulates the system with two frequencies, $\omega_1$ and $\omega_2$, simultaneously, say with

$$B \, Sin(\omega_1 t) + C \, Sin(\omega_2 t), \tag{3}$$

then the response will look like

$$R(t) = A(\omega_1) \, B \, Sin(\omega_1 t) + A(\omega_2) \, C \, Sin(\omega_2 t). \tag{4}$$

You can see a trend here. This is just the sum of the responses of the system when it is being driven at each frequency separately. This is also what is meant by linear. The equation shows that the response has two frequencies present and these are precisely the frequencies at which the system is being driven. The only difference is that their amplitudes are affected differently depending on the frequency response of the system. Doubling the amplitude of one of the stimulation frequencies will result in a doubling of the response amplitude at that frequency only.

At this point you should take a moment and make sure it is clear to you that the response in equation (4) consists of two frequencies, $\omega_1$ and $\omega_2$. Just read the equation and look at the sine functions that are being summed. There is one sine wave of frequency $\omega_1$ plus one sine wave of frequency $\omega_2$. Note that the sine waves could be replaced with cosines and one would still obtain the same frequencies. This is because a sine wave is a phase-shifted version of a cosine wave.

## QUADRATIC NONLINEARITIES

Not all systems have to work like this. What happens if the presence of two frequencies in the driving stimulus affects the response differently than described above? Consider the following response function:

$$R(t) = A(\omega_1) \, B \, Sin(\omega_1 t) + A(\omega_2) \, C \, Sin(\omega_2 t) + D(\omega_1, \omega_2) \, B \, Sin(\omega_1 t) \, C \, Sin(\omega_2 t). \qquad (5)$$

It is the same as before, but now there is a third term that depends on the product of the two driving sine waves and a new frequency response function, $D(\omega_1, \omega_2)$, that depends on both driving frequencies.

Things are getting a little messy so let's simplify a bit. Say that the frequency response of the system in all cases is $A(\omega) = 1$ and that $D(\omega_1, \omega_2) = 1$. In addition, let's say that the driving stimuli have unit amplitude so that $B = 1$ and $C = 1$. This strips away the unnecessary detail so we can better visualize what is happening. The simplified response becomes

$$R(t) = Sin(\omega_1 t) + Sin(\omega_2 t) + Sin(\omega_1 t) \, Sin(\omega_2 t). \qquad (6)$$

This response depends on the sum of the sine functions at the two driving frequencies and the product of those sine functions. There is no reason that this cannot happen physically, and in fact, complications like this are quite common in approximations of real systems. The last term is called a nonlinear term.

There are several similar nonlinear terms that we could have added (note that 7b is the one above):

$$Sin(\omega_1 t) \, Sin(\omega_1 t) = Sin^2(\omega_1 t) \qquad (7a)$$
$$Sin(\omega_1 t) \, Sin(\omega_2 t) \qquad (7b)$$
$$Sin(\omega_2 t) \, Sin(\omega_2 t) = Sin^2(\omega_2 t) \qquad (7c)$$

These terms have the effect of destroying the linearity of the response. If the amplitude of one of the driving frequencies is doubled, then the response at that frequency is not necessarily doubled. In addition, the response at one frequency may now depend on the response at another frequency. This is called nonlinearity and the system is said to be nonlinear. More specifically, as the nonlinear term consists of the product of two sine functions, the nonlinearity is said to be quadratic (as computing the area of a square or quadrilateral requires the product of two terms, the height and the width). Another example is the quadratic equation, $a \, x^2 + b \, x + c = 0$, where the x squared term is a nonlinear term similar to (7a) above. Nonlinearities often imply interactions among the components of the system. In this case, the responses to the two driving oscillations are interacting with one another.

In this simple nonlinear system, what frequencies are found in the response? Well, the response is

$$R(t) = Sin(\omega_1 t) + Sin(\omega_2 t) + Sin(\omega_1 t) \, Sin(\omega_2 t). \qquad (6)$$

It looks like we have an $\omega_1$ from the first sine function and an $\omega_2$ from the second sine function, but the third quadratic term is not a simple sine wave so we cannot just read off the frequencies. We need to do some trigonometry. One can look up the following trigonometric identities (one can also derive these writing the sine waves in terms of exponentials):

$$\text{Sin}(A)\,\text{Sin}(B) \;=\; \tfrac{1}{2}\,[\,\text{Cos}(A - B) - \text{Cos}(A + B)\,] \tag{I1}$$

$$\text{Cos}(A)\,\text{Cos}(B) \;=\; \tfrac{1}{2}\,[\,\text{Cos}(A - B) + \text{Cos}(A + B)\,] \tag{I2}$$

$$\text{Sin}(A)\,\text{Cos}(B) \;=\; \tfrac{1}{2}\,[\,\text{Sin}(A - B) + \text{Sin}(A + B)\,] \tag{I3}$$

$$\text{Cos}(A - B) \;=\; \text{Cos}(B - A) \tag{I4}$$

$$\text{Sin}(A - B) \;=\; -\text{Sin}(B - A) \tag{I5}$$

The first three identities describe how products of sines and cosines are related to sums of sines and cosines. This will be useful in evaluating our product of sine functions. The last two identities describe the symmetry of the sine and cosine functions. You can probably see where this is going. We can use identity (I1) above to deal with our product of sine functions and we will get a sum of cosines. Let's try it. First just look at the third term in the response (6) and use identity (I1) above:

$$\text{Sin}(\omega_1 t)\,\text{Sin}(\omega_2 t) = \tfrac{1}{2}\,[\,\text{Cos}(\omega_1 t - \omega_2 t) - \text{Cos}(\omega_1 t + \omega_2 t)\,] \tag{8}$$

Since, usually $\omega_2 > \omega_1$, we can rewrite the first cosine, $\text{Cos}(\omega_1 t - \omega_2 t)$, using identity (I4) and get $\text{Cos}(\omega_2 t - \omega_1 t)$. We can also factor out the t's writing $(\omega_2 t - \omega_1 t)$ as $((\omega_2 - \omega_1)\,t)$, and do the same for $(\omega_1 t + \omega_2 t)$. The result is

$$\text{Sin}(\omega_1 t)\,\text{Sin}(\omega_2 t) = \tfrac{1}{2}\,[\,\text{Cos}((\omega_2 - \omega_1)t) - \text{Cos}((\omega_1 + \omega_2)t)\,]. \tag{9}$$

Finally, the response function in equation (6) can be rewritten as

$$R(t) = \text{Sin}(\omega_1 t) + \text{Sin}(\omega_2 t) + \tfrac{1}{2}\,\text{Cos}((\omega_2 - \omega_1)t) - \tfrac{1}{2}\,\text{Cos}((\omega_1 + \omega_2)t). \tag{10}$$

You should follow along with pencil and paper to make sure you get the idea. Now we have a sum of sines and cosines and we can read off the angular frequencies present in the response. These frequencies are $\omega_1$, $\omega_2$, $(\omega_2 - \omega_1)$, and $(\omega_1 + \omega_2)$. Replacing $\omega$ with $2\pi f$ we find that the frequencies present in the response are $f_1$, $f_2$, $(f_2 - f_1)$, $(f_1 + f_2)$. We have derived the quadratic distortion products $(f_2 - f_1)$ and $(f_1 + f_2)$. Remember that they come from the quadratic nonlinearity in the response function and are due to an interaction between the responses to both frequencies. For this reason, they are called quadratic distortion products. Note also that their contribution to the response is only one half as much as the linear terms. They are generally not as strong as the responses to the two original frequencies. If you are wondering why sines and cosines are both present in the response, remember that a cosine is a phase-shifted sine wave and vice versa. In addition, the negative amplitude of a sine or cosine can also be interpreted as a phase-shift, as in the fourth term in equation (10) above. I have done my best to keep phase effects out of this tutorial, but in some cases, it is unavoidable.

## CUBIC NONLINEARITIES

As you may have already guessed, the response of the system can be even more complicated. Let's look at a response like this:

$$R(t) = Sin(\omega_1 t) + Sin(\omega_2 t) + Sin^2(\omega_1 t)\, Sin(\omega_2 t) \tag{11}$$

where the third term can be written as $Sin(\omega_1 t)\, Sin(\omega_1 t)\, Sin(\omega_2 t)$. It is a product of three sine functions and is called a cubic nonlinearity. The terminology comes from the fact that the volume of a cube is the product of three quantities, its length, its width, and its height.

What is the frequency content of this response? Well, again we can easily read off the frequencies from the first two terms, $\omega_1$ and $\omega_2$, but the third term again isn't a pure sine or cosine function. We have to expand the cubic term into a sum of sines and cosines again. To expand this let's look at the $Sin^2(\omega_1 t)$ part first. Using identity (I1) again (this is the same as before, but now A and B are both equal to $\omega_1$):

$$
\begin{aligned}
Sin(\omega_1 t)\, Sin(\omega_1 t) &= \tfrac{1}{2}\,[\, Cos((\omega_1 - \omega_1)t) - Cos((\omega_1 + \omega_1)t)\,] \\
&= \tfrac{1}{2}\,[\, Cos(0) - Cos(2\omega_1 t)\,] \\
&= \tfrac{1}{2}\,[\, 1 - Cos(2\omega_1 t)\,] \\
&= [\, \tfrac{1}{2} - \tfrac{1}{2} Cos(2\omega_1 t)\,]. \tag{15}
\end{aligned}
$$

Substituting equation (15) into the cubic term in equation (11) we find that

$$Sin^2(\omega_1 t)\, Sin(\omega_2 t) = [\, \tfrac{1}{2} - \tfrac{1}{2} Cos(2\omega_1 t)\,]\, Sin(\omega_2 t). \tag{16}$$

We continue using the same procedure as before. Any time we see a product of sines and cosines we use the identities above to turn them into sums of sines or cosines.

$$\text{Sin}^2(\omega_1 t) \, \text{Sin}(\omega_2 t) = [\, \tfrac{1}{2} - \tfrac{1}{2} \text{Cos}(2\omega_1 t)\,] \, \text{Sin}(\omega_2 t)$$
$$= \tfrac{1}{2} \text{Sin}(\omega_2 t) - \tfrac{1}{2} \text{Cos}(2\omega_1 t) \, \text{Sin}(\omega_2 t)$$
$$= \tfrac{1}{2} \text{Sin}(\omega_2 t) - \tfrac{1}{2} \text{Sin}(\omega_2 t) \, \text{Cos}(2\omega_1 t) \tag{17}$$

Now that we have multiplied it out, there is now a product of a sine and a cosine so we can use identity (I3) to expand it into a sum of sines:

$$= \tfrac{1}{2} \text{Sin}(\omega_2 t) - \tfrac{1}{2} \{\, \tfrac{1}{2} [\, \text{Sin}(\omega_2 t - 2\omega_1 t) + \text{Sin}(\omega_2 t + 2\omega_1 t)]\}$$
$$= \tfrac{1}{2} \text{Sin}(\omega_2 t) - \tfrac{1}{4} \text{Sin}(\omega_2 t - 2\omega_1 t) - \tfrac{1}{4} \text{Sin}(\omega_2 t + 2\omega_1 t). \tag{18}$$

Recall that we can use identity (I5) to set $\text{Sin}(\omega_2 t - 2\omega_1 t) = -\text{Sin}(2\omega_1 t - \omega_2 t)$, and we know that $\text{Sin}(\omega_2 t + 2\omega_1 t) = \text{Sin}(2\omega_1 t + \omega_2 t)$ so we get

$$= \tfrac{1}{2} \text{Sin}(\omega_2 t) + \tfrac{1}{4} \text{Sin}(2\omega_1 t - \omega_2 t) - \tfrac{1}{4} \text{Sin}(2\omega_1 t + \omega_2 t)$$
$$= \tfrac{1}{2} \text{Sin}(\omega_2 t) + \tfrac{1}{4} \text{Sin}(2\omega_1 - \omega_2)t) - \tfrac{1}{4} \text{Sin}((2\omega_1 + \omega_2)t). \tag{19}$$

Now we can put the expanded cubic term above (19) back into the response equation (11),

$$R(t) = \text{Sin}(\omega_1 t) + \text{Sin}(\omega_2 t) + \tfrac{1}{2} \text{Sin}(\omega_2 t) + \tfrac{1}{4} \text{Sin})(2\omega_1 - \omega_2)t) - \tfrac{1}{4} \text{Sin}((2\omega_1 + \omega_2)t), \tag{20}$$

and simplify it by combining the second and third terms to obtain our result:

$$R(t) = \text{Sin}(\omega_1 t) + \tfrac{3}{2} \text{Sin}(\omega_2 t) + \tfrac{1}{4} \text{Sin}((2\omega_1 - \omega_2)t) - \tfrac{1}{4} \text{Sin}((2\omega_1 + \omega_2)t). \tag{21}$$

Now we can read off the angular frequencies found in the response. We find $\omega_1$, $\omega_2$, $(2\omega_1 - \omega_2)$, and $(2\omega_1 + \omega_2)$, which correspond to the frequencies $f_1$, $f_2$, $(2f_1 - f_2)$, and $(2f_1 + f_2)$. We have found the cubic distortion products $(2f_1 - f_2)$ and $(2f_1 + f_2)$. Notice that these frequencies are only one fourth of the amplitude of the responses of the original driving frequencies. This is an interesting trend. The higher order interactions generally produce lower amplitude distortion products. In addition to the new frequencies, the amplitude of $f_2$ in this case is increased to $\tfrac{3}{2}$ because of the extra signal at $f_2$ produced by the distortion product. This is another way that these nonlinearities can appear.

## RELATION TO REAL OTOACOUSTIC EMISSIONS

We have just worked through two examples of nonlinear responses where we encountered the quadratic distortion product, $(f_2 - f_1)$, and the cubic distortion product, $(2f_1 - f_2)$, common in otoacoustic emissions. One may wonder why the other products derived are not readily seen in otoacoustic emissions. We must remember that we have simplified the problem in the analysis above by neglecting the frequency response of the system. In addition, there may be higher order effects that cancel out some of the lower order distortion products, in a way opposite of the enhancement of the $\omega_2$ term above in equation (21). The model responses that we have been playing with are by no means an accurate portrayal of the otoacoustic responses in the auditory system. Something like

$$R(t) = \text{Sin}(\omega_1 t) + \text{Sin}(\omega_2 t) + \text{Sin}(\omega_1 t)\,\text{Sin}(\omega_2 t) + \text{Sin}^2(\omega_1 t)\,\text{Sin}(\omega_2 t) \tag{22}$$

may be a good first guess. It predicts frequencies $f_1$, $f_2$, $(f_2 - f_1)$, $(f_2 + f_1)$, $(2f_1 - f_2)$, and $(2f_1 + f_2)$. Why should the sine function, $\text{Sin}(\omega_1 t)$, in the cubic term be preferred (by squaring) over $\text{Sin}(\omega_2 t)$? Maybe the response should be made symmetric with respect to $\omega_1$ and $\omega_2$, like this:

$$R(t) = \text{Sin}(\omega_1 t) + \text{Sin}(\omega_2 t) + \text{Sin}(\omega_1 t)\,\text{Sin}(\omega_2 t) + \text{Sin}^2(\omega_1 t)\,\text{Sin}(\omega_2 t) + \text{Sin}(\omega_1 t)\,\text{Sin}^2(\omega_2 t). \tag{23}$$

Perhaps one should include all the combinations:

$$R(t) = \text{Sin}(\omega_1 t) + \text{Sin}(\omega_2 t) + \qquad\qquad\text{(Linear Terms)}$$
$$\text{Sin}^2(\omega_1 t) + \text{Sin}(\omega_1 t)\,\text{Sin}(\omega_2 t) + \text{Sin}^2(\omega_2 t) + \qquad\text{(Quadratic Terms)}$$
$$\text{Sin}^3(\omega_1 t) + \text{Sin}^2(\omega_1 t)\,\text{Sin}(\omega_2 t) + \text{Sin}(\omega_1 t)\,\text{Sin}^2(\omega_2 t) + \text{Sin}^3(\omega_2 t) \ \text{(Cubic Terms)}. \tag{24}$$

What happens in this case? (This one you can work out yourself to test your understanding.)

In a more realistic model, the terms can have different amplitudes, and these amplitudes should depend on the frequencies. Therefore, depending on the system, some distortion products will be strong whereas others will be weak or even cancel out! Try the next one in equation (25). The results are surprising.

$$R(t) = 2\,\text{Sin}(\omega_1 t) - \tfrac{1}{2}\,\text{Sin}(\omega_2 t) + \text{Sin}^2(\omega_1 t)\,\text{Sin}(\omega_2 t). \tag{25}$$

It is similar to the cubic case that we just worked through, but this time one of the original frequencies doesn't even appear in the response!

## A BIT FURTHER

What happens when there are quartic, or fourth-order terms, such as $\text{Sin}^4(\omega_1 t)$ or $\text{Sin}^2(\omega_1 t)\,\text{Sin}^2(\omega_2 t)$? Try working them out. For the first one treat the $\text{Sin}^4(\omega_1 t)$ as $\text{Sin}^2(\omega_1 t)\,\text{Sin}^2(\omega_1 t)$ and use identity (I1) to expand each quadratic term separately. Then multiply the expanded terms out to get quadratic terms with cosines. Expand these quadratic terms and you'll have the answer. The second example can be solved similarly.

One can show that any nonlinear term will result in frequencies of the form $| n_1 f_1 + n_2 f_2 |$, where $n_1$ and $n_2$ are integers and the bars signify that one should take the absolute value (this avoids negative frequencies). Also, if $n_1 + n_2$ is even, then the nonlinearity is an even order (like the quadratic), and if $n_1 + n_2$ is odd, then the nonlinearity is an odd order (like the cubic).

Another interesting result is that if the ratio of the two driving frequencies, $f_1/f_2$, is rational (i.e., $f_1/f_2 = p/q$, where p and q are integers), then all of the frequencies in the response must be multiples or harmonics of $f_2 - f_1$. If the ratio of the frequencies is irrational, then $| n_1 f_1 + n_2 f_2 |$ can produce all possible frequencies. It is important to remember that although all frequencies might be present in the response, the spectrum will not be smooth and continuous. Nearby frequencies may have very different amplitudes.

How do the amplitudes of the frequencies, $| n_1 f_1 + n_2 f_2 |$, behave as $n_1$ or $n_2$ becomes large (for example when we have $| 5f_1 + 7f_2 |$)? Well, as we saw above, the quadratic term in the response function resulted in $|n| = 1$ and the amplitudes were only ½. The cubic term resulted in $|n_i| = 1$ and $|n_j| = 2$, and the amplitudes were decreased to ¼. Generally, the amplitudes of the frequencies follow $\text{Exp}( -a_1 |n_1| - a_2 |n_2| )$, where $a_1$ and $a_2$ are positive numbers depending on the nonlinearity. As $|n_1|$ and $|n_2|$ get large, specifically as soon as $|n_1|$ and $|n_2|$ exceed $a_1^{-1}$ and $a_2^{-1}$, the amplitude of the corresponding frequency becomes negligibly small and cannot be detected (Bergé, Pomeau, & Vidal, 1984).

We have looked at what can happen with the occurrence of two frequencies in the driving stimulus, but we have not considered interactions among three or more frequencies. As you might guess, there will be more distortion products. Specifically if r frequencies are presented, the observed frequencies will be of the form $| n_1 f_1 + n_2 f_2 + n_3 f_3 + \ldots + n_r f_r |$. If the ratio of any pair of frequencies is irrational, then all frequencies can be present in the response. If all of the ratios are rational, the response will consist of multiples or harmonics of the differences between all of the pairs of driving frequencies.

We have not considered what happens with the phases of the responses. This matter is much more complicated. If we stimulate a linear system at a certain driving frequency then the system will oscillate at that frequency. The phase of the system's oscillation depends on the resonance frequency of the system, the damping in the system, and the driving frequency. For a system with nonlinearities, the phase becomes more difficult to deal with and we will not discuss the topic in this tutorial. In the context of otoacoustic emissions, this becomes even more difficult as the travel time between the source of the emissions and the recording microphone will introduce an additional phase shift. The presence of multiple emission sites would further complicate the calculation of the phase of the response.

## CONCLUSION

When a linear system is simultaneously driven at multiple frequencies, it will respond only at those frequencies. However, nonlinearities in the system, which can be described as interactions among the responses to the various frequencies present in the driving stimulus, will cause the system to respond at frequencies not necessarily present in the driving stimulus. These new frequencies are called distortion products. A quadratic nonlinearity will cause a quadratic distortion product, a cubic nonlinearity will cause a cubic distortion product, and so on. These nonlinearities can also affect the response amplitudes at the original driving frequencies. As we have seen, the distortion products are a result of the presence of nonlinearities in oscillations in general and are not restricted to biological phenomena. Therefore, one should expect that under certain conditions microphones and transducers used in the acquisition of otoacoustic emissions can generate distortion products. This occurs when they are driven outside of their linear operating range into a regime where the device behaves nonlinearly. This is an important fact to consider when performing distortion product otoacoustic emission experiments. One must be sure that the distortion products are due to the physiology of the inner ear of the subject and not due to the equipment.

Distortion products can provide much information about the nonlinearities present in a system. Although it is important to remember that a single system can produce quadratic, cubic, quartic, and higher order distortion products simultaneously, it is also important to note that there are sometimes different components of a system that are producing similar or different distortion products. For example, the presence of quadratic and cubic distortion products in an otoacoustic emission experiment does not imply that there are necessarily two distortion product sources present. One physical effect may produce both types of distortion products simultaneously. In addition, experimental manipulation of the system can change the frequency response of the system and thus affect the various orders of distortion products differently. For this reason, one must be careful not to assume that the distortion products of different orders originate from distinct sources solely on the basis that the variation of one variable in the experiment affected the distortion products differently. However, there is no reason to assume, a priori, that there is one source of nonlinearity in the inner ear. Basilar membrane motion, inner and outer hair cell motion, and efferent effects can possibly all contribute to the observed distortion products.

**Acknowledgments:** This work was supported by Kam's Fund for Hearing Research, the Kresge Hearing Research Laboratory, and NIH NIDCD 5 T32 DC00007.

## REFERENCES

Bergé, P., Pomeau, Y., & Vidal, C. (1984). *Order within chaos: Towards a deterministic approach to turbulence.* New York: John Wiley & Sons.

Lins, O. G., & Picton, T. W. (1995). Auditory steady-state responses to multiple simultaneous stimuli. *Electroencephalography and Clinical Neurophysiology, 96,* 420–432.

# Index

# Echoes of the Travelling Wave CD-Rom

*David T. Kemp, Ph.D.*

The CD-ROM enclosed in this book contains the following three programs:

DIEP1D: a working demonstration of Cochlear Travelling Waves

REALTIME: this program can collect and display actual OAEs in realtime in conjunction with any ILO-compatible hardware

ILOV55: this program can load and view many OAE example files and perform analysis. It can also simulate OAE recording sessions on computers that do not have ILO-compatible hardware.

## INSTALLATION

RUN INSTALL on the CD ROM. This will install the Travelling Wave and REALTIME OAE program into directory C:\OAEWAVES Run the programs by double clicking on the DIEP1D or REALTIME icons on your desktop or by running the programs by name. Disk requirement is less then 1 megabyte

The program ILOV5 can be run from the CD Rom without installation and is NOT "installed" automatically. Certain functions cannot be run from CD, and it may be manually installed on the hard drive if demonstration of DPOAEs are required.

DO NOT install ILOV5 on your hard drive if you already have an ILO-compatible system installed. To install and run ILOV5 on the hard drive:

Assuming your CD is the D: drive then run the MSDOS prompt and key in the following instructions pressing Enter after each line

1) CD\
2) MD ILO-V5
3) CD ILO-V5
4) XCOPY D:\ILO-V5\*.*/S
5) COPY D:\ILOV5.BAT
6) ILOV5

## RUNNING THE PROGRAMS

After installation in Windows 95, Icons will appear on the desktop names DIEP1D and REALTIME. Double click on these to run the programs. If no Icons appear, go to RUN, Browse C:\OAEWAVES and select DIEP1D or REALTIME to run

To run ILOV5 from the CD Start MSDOS prompt, select the CD drive e.g., d: and type ILOV5 and enter.

## USING THE PROGRAMS

DIEP1D offers three choices

1) Travelling waves—the animation can be paused and cochlear parameters changed as per instructions on screen
2) This is a static screen shot of a TEOAE waveform—no menu options are available
3) This is a static screen shot of a DPOAE waveform—no menu options are available

REALTIME looks for ILO-compatible hardware in your PC. Select the type you have.

Use cursor up and down to adjust noise artifact rejection, and Page Up and Down to alter screen scales. Save OAE waveforms to the lower panel with S key. With strong OAEs and a quiet room, clear, repeatable OAEs will be seen in in realtime. When the trace goes red—it means there is noise rejection. Green means acoustic data are being recorded and analyzed. The program cannot be run without ILO hardware.

ILOV5 shows an "IL088" introductory screen. Press Enter and select the TEOAE box with mouse or T. Select Files, Review to list examples. Enter to load and select. F3 for spectrum and F5 for cursor. H for half octave analysis. Once an example is loaded, a simulated test can be run. Select Test Quickscreen. Enter patient name n99 for noise patient. Press Enter two times to start the test running. Adjust noise rejection with Up/Down keys.

Some menu options will cause the program to halt, because they require to write information on the disk. This is not possible with a CD. See above for hard disk operation.

If installed on the hard drive, you may select Tests DPOAE for distortion product program. In this program Files Load will list examples. Test DPgram will run a simulated DPOAE recording. All menus operate. The DP demonstration is not active when run from the CD

## REMOVAL

To remove DIEP1D and REALTIME, delete directory C:\OAEWAVES from the C: prompt with deltree c:\oaewaves or from Windows explorer. To remove Icons, right click on the Icon and chose delete.

To remove ILOV5 if this has been manually copied from disk, delete directory c:\lLO-V5. DO NOT remove ILO-V5 from systems actually installed with ILO hardware.